Mindfulness for Brain Health

Neuroscience-Informed Mindfulness in Plain English, Empowering You with Self-Care and Mindfulness Meditation Practices for Clarity, Peace and Joy

Dr Sui H. Wong MD FRCP

EBH Press. EBHpress.com. Copyright © 2024 Dr Sui H. Wong.

ISBN: 978-1-7385581-1-7 (Paperback) 978-1-7385581-0-0 (E-book)

978-1-7385581-0-0 (Hardcover), 978-1-917353-23-6 (Audiobook)

"Dr Wong reframes mindfulness from the spiritual to the scientific. This book provides a no-nonsense practical guide to improve both mental and neurological health, demonstrating the medical benefits of this technique for all aspects of our wellbeing."
~ Prof. Guy Leschziner, Professor of Neurology and Sleep Medicine

"At last - the definitive guide to Mindfulness based on how our brains really work, written in everyday language by a world leading expert in brain science. If you want to be truly happy – read this book!"
~ David Taylor, Author of The Naked Leader best-selling books,
Global Business Ambassador The Kings Trust,
Visiting Professor The Open University

Table of Contents

This book is dedicated to my mother and late father.

The Science of Mindfulness

Do you ever have days when you feel dissatisfied with your life? Days when that critical inner voice says, "You're not good enough"? Do you find yourself making comparisons with other people, friends, family or work colleagues, thinking they seem to have aced life? *Why can't you be like that?*

Social media hasn't helped this, giving us a heavily filtered window into the lives of others. This doesn't just impact children and teenagers; it affects all age groups. When we constantly see polished photos and videos of what other people are doing, it can be hard to remember that what other people do might not translate into our own lives. Plus, what we're seeing is just a snapshot - a moment in time.

You might feel like you're the only person who does this, but the truth is, you're not alone. We're all geared towards social comparison. Contextualising ourselves in societal groups is part of how we create our sense of self-definition. It helps us answer some of those core questions we have about ourselves: Who am I? Who do I want to be? But this is only valuable to a certain degree. Constant negative comparisons can lead to dissatisfaction, feelings of inadequacy and become harmful to our emotional health over time.

As I reflect on my journey to becoming a neurologist, I realize that achieving success, particularly in competitive fields like medicine, often fosters a mindset of scarcity. In my pursuit of admission to medical school, I strived to excel academically, driven by the perception of limited spots available. I was also a worrier. This mindset led me to adopt a comparison-oriented approach, constantly measuring myself against others, and worrying about negative outcomes. I've come to recognize the detrimental effects of this mindset and have actively worked to cultivate self-compassion and kindness.

Now, I'm passionate about exploring the impact of mindset on well-being, both in my professional practice and in my personal life. Rather than perpetuating the cycle of comparison, worrying and overthinking, I strive to promote a culture of generosity, self-compassion and understanding. Through my work, I aim to empower others to embrace kindness towards themselves and others, recognizing that true success is not measured by comparison, but by inner fulfilment and genuine connection.

How can those of us who are overthinkers find more peace, be less self-critical and feel less overwhelmed? And what benefits for brain health might we uncover in the process? It was on this journey that I discovered mindfulness.

The power of mindfulness for our brains forms the heart of this book. I'm excited to share this journey with you and hope as you read through the chapters ahead, you'll find the answers you've been looking for to the questions above and much more.

What Holds Us Back

If you frequently consider ways of making positive changes to your life or seek improvements in a certain practice you've started, you are not alone in this quest. We can all understand the principle, but it's not until we get in amongst it that we find out just how hard it can be.

The reality of the human condition is that change is often intimidating and it's not unusual to feel bored or distracted, uneasy or confused. We all want quick results, a quick fix so it's very easy to lose heart or become frustrated and give up when the going gets a bit tough. Sound familiar? Just think how many New Year's resolutions are in the bin by the end of January! However, persistence really does have its rewards.

I'll give you a relatable example of how much power the mind can have over a person. Running was my nemesis 30 years ago. I wanted to make running part of my fitness routine, take on the challenge to run half or full marathons. I was horrified when I went on my first run, that I couldn't even run one block without having to stop to catch my breath. I knew I needed to build my endurance in running, so I followed a program that tracked my heart rate and allowed me to build my stamina over time. On many days, I found this way of training tedious. With the program I had chosen, I had to keep to a slow pace to build my stamina, but at the pace I was running, anyone next to me could pass me by at a brisk walk.

I got frustrated with my slow progress. *Why is this so hard for me?* I'd think to myself. *Will I ever be able to run a mile, let alone a marathon?* These thoughts only made my mind more frustrated and stressed with my lack of progress.

One day, after weeks of feeling like I wasn't improving, I found myself focusing on the way I breathed in and out during my run. This was years before I even knew what mindfulness training was, so I wasn't quite sure what I was doing, but I found that focusing on the sensation of each step as I breathed in and out allowed me to set a steady and manageable pace as I ran. As I focused on my breath, I also found my mind remained within the moment, allowing my breath and the pace of my steps to guide me. I found that this helped me to become more relaxed and in the moment as I ran.

While running may not be one of your mental blocks in life, I'm going to guess that some activity causes you to feel anxious or stressed when you think about it, and the more you fixate on this activity, the more troubled you become. So often, we think about certain conversations we dread, daily chores we don't want to complete, or nerve-racking experiences we worry about participating in. These feelings are natural since we all overthink at some point in our lives but, when this happens, we have two choices. We can either dwell on these ideas and travel down a road of feeling worse, or we can do something about it and learn to deal with our emotions with calmness and composure. The key to doing the latter can be unlocked with the practice of mindfulness.

Mindfulness and Neuroplasticity

While learning to stay mindful may not make us fall in love with the tasks that we don't want to do, this practice can create more of a relaxed state of being within our minds so that we can have a comfortable perception of our surroundings. This change allows us to become an observer of any problems or anxious thoughts we're having rather than remaining a vulnerable participant in a miserable experience that doesn't serve us well.

So, what is this seemingly remarkable idea that can lead to more fulfilling experiences in life? While the idea of mindfulness has a variety of meanings for different individuals, the concept mainly boils down to creating an awareness of an experience. So often, we associate mindfulness solely with the practice of meditation and a "clearing of the mind," but it's so much more than that. Instead of thinking about nothing or trying to clear the mind completely, which is nearly impossible, practicing mindfulness offers us the chance to stay present in our current moment and to act as an observer of our thoughts.

There's no denying that practicing how to create a state of mindfulness is difficult. For many, the idea of taking the time to slow down or add another practice to their already busy schedule just doesn't feel feasible. This sounds valid when you think about mindfulness as a separate activity that you have to add to your day, but when you think of it as connected to everything you do, it becomes a more realistic pursuit.

In studies of the brain, scientists have found viewable changes that occur in brain matter as a direct result of a person learning to practice mindfulness, specifically with a meditation practice. In one study, scientists concluded that even a short-term practice of mindfulness can alter the brain's ability for increased conflict resolution and emotional control (Tang et al., 2012). Since neuroplasticity, or brain plasticity, means that our brains are capable of changing to adapt or respond to internal and external stimuli, the mindful practices we incorporate can have lasting effects on our perception (Puderbaugh & Emmady, 2023).

Popular Mindfulness

Have you noticed that the idea of mindfulness and self-care seems to have seeped into our world even more over the last decade? The growing interest in how to become more calm and stress-free over the last ten to twenty years is no coincidence.

So, why is mindfulness so popular as a practice now? While researchers have many theories to answer this question, they've reached several top conclusions. The most prominent seems to relate to the fast-growing stress that society faces daily, the destigmatization of mental health issues, and more promising scientific evidence that mindful practices are beneficial for brain health (Bernstein et al., 2019). While it can be disheartening to know that stressful circumstances have warranted the popularity of a practice, you can take comfort in the fact that, with its benefits and destigmatization, the incorporation of mindfulness in schools, workplaces, and general culture will continue to benefit this booming practice.

My Passion for Mindfulness

Let me take a moment now to introduce myself. I have long been fascinated by the functions and mysteries of the human brain. As a neurologist and neuro-ophthalmologist, I work with patients who have a range of conditions, and I've dedicated over twenty years of my life to neurology and neuroscience. While physicians and scientists are learning more in this field every day, my research has led me to see just how impactful the practice of mindfulness is for a patient's treatment and care. In addition to my medical training, I've completed training as a hypnotherapist and I've found a passion for teaching yoga and mindfulness to others.

I have been dedicated to bring mindfulness into the medical and neurological setting, through good quality research. As part of this passion and dedication, I have led and delivered clinical research trials with mindfulness as a treatment intervention for neurological conditions, and continue to work tirelessly in this area to improve patient outcomes.

My goal as a physician, researcher, and writer is to empower others with quality information that will help them enhance their well-being. In my clinical practice, I often see patients who are unaware of the actionable steps they can take to improve their health both physically and mentally. I also meet with many patients who seem confused about the benefits that a mindful practice can offer.

Although I have written many academic research papers and book chapters, this is my first book for the public. My mission as I venture into this new world of writing books for the public, is to share good quality actionable information to benefit your brain health and wellbeing.

This book will help beginners who are interested in mindfulness, to successfully introduce this into their daily lives. My goal here, is to provide you with useful, actionable, and practical information to facilitate the implementation of this practice. For those interested, I have also shared the benefits of mindfulness through a neuroscientific lens.

This book is your resource for easy to use and immediately available practices for improved mindfulness. To further enhance and embed your practice, you could consider this as part of your "year of mindfulness" with easy-to-follow mindful and self-care ideas, that will help you feel both calm and motivated on your path to wellbeing.

The ideas offered at the end of Chapters 1 through 12 will allow you to get started immediately, by preparing the grounds for a mindful path through self-care approaches. With this guide, you have suggestions you can pull from for each month of the year. You could even try incorporating a new one each day or week during your "year of mindfulness."

While the ideas included in each chapter may not feel revolutionary, they're meant to be simple, practical methods to start you on your development of a more open and positive mind.

These self-care ideas can settle your body and mind, so you can incorporate mindfulness into your life consistently. These are even simple enough that you could begin incorporating certain ideas today to kick-start a more mindful existence.

You may find it helpful to use this book alongside guided mindfulness practices such as breathing meditations, breathwork, body scan, and movement practices. I cover these in the relevant chapters in the book, and signpost to audioguides which you an access with this book.

I hope you find this book enjoyable and helpful.

"The journey of a thousand miles begins with a single step"
– Lao Tzu

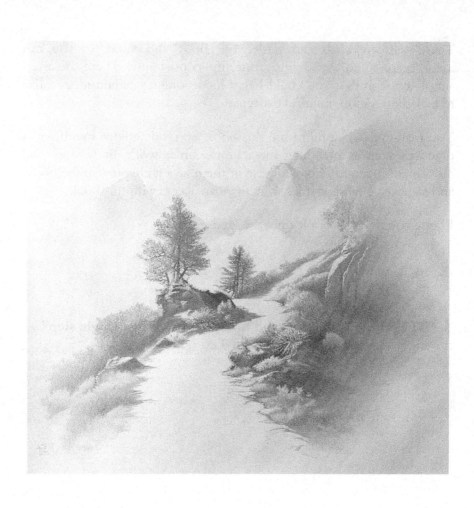

Chapter 1:

Exploring Neuroplasticity

Have you ever witnessed a toddler in full meltdown mode? I'm talking kicking and screaming on the ground because something isn't going their way. In moments like these, do you ever think to yourself, *There are days when I feel like doing that, too?*

While adults tend to possess the ability to restrain physical meltdowns in life, our anxious behaviors seep out in other ways if we don't cultivate a helpful approach to handling stressors.

For example, a busy parent who works ten-hour days and still has to make dinner for their family, pack lunches for their children for the next school day, and study for an online course at night might find their moods fluctuating more than usual throughout their day because of how many activities they're juggling. This parent may feel stressed, angry, and even argumentative as a result of their packed schedule, and understandably so.

Regulating our feelings becomes a challenge when we jump from one activity to the next day after day. If you have a chance, slow down for a few moments after a busy day. What does this feel like? For many, their minds may still be racing from the momentum of what they've experienced up until that moment, leading to an inability to relax. A person's mind may wander to their to-do list or to a mistake they find themselves fixating on from earlier in the day.

Some try to combat life's never-ending busyness with vices such as coffee, alcohol, drugs, or wasting money on unneeded items, but doing this tends to provide only temporary relief from any stress we're experiencing. There is another approach to living that doesn't require any expensive equipment, gym memberships, or negative habits to create a better sense of self and well-being. It lies in our ability to reshape our brains.

Important Brain Signals

Let's face it—our brains try to do more than we sometimes want them to. If you've ever experienced a racing mind at night when you just want to sleep, you know what I'm talking about. Because of the brain's complexities and functions, it wants to make sense of situations and organize thoughts into categories in our minds at most moments of the day. How helpful, right? Whilst this ability is amazing for problem-solving and quick decision-making, it's not as great when we want to relax but are unable to "switch off" constant thinking.

Our brain is constantly working behind the scenes to make sure that messages are sent and connections are made so that we interpret and process information correctly. The signals our brain sends breathe life into our muscle movement, sight, hearing, smell, taste, and touch.

The vital meeting place for communication in our brains is known as the synapse, which is an area that releases chemical signals called neurotransmitters (Sivadas & Broadie, 2020). "One of the most important things about our brains is that synapses change when we use them. These changes in our synapses (plasticity) allow us to learn new information, and then remember what we have learned" (Sivadas & Broadie, 2020). It's through these signals that our mind forms memories that will help us throughout life.

Without these synapses, we'd have to relearn the steps of the daily tasks we perform from the beginning every time we try to do them. Of course, when the brain is altered if it experiences an injury like a stroke, concussion, or burst aneurysm, synapse messages may have difficulty completing their job. The plasticity of our brains allows for either beneficial or negative changes to occur, which is why incorporating mindful practices into our lives can allow our brain networks to change in the best way possible.

Embracing the Practice

If you've felt hesitant to incorporate more mindful practices in your own life because you don't believe you have enough time or because you simply can't imagine the value it will provide, consider the following. Mindfulness practices don't necessarily have to be something that a person takes time out of their day to do separately. Instead, the mindful activities one performs are meant to enhance every aspect of a person's day by bringing enhanced concentration, clarity, and peacefulness to all situations. As with anything, there will be hard days and easy days with mindfulness at first.. Think of mindfulness as an ongoing lifestyle practice.

While incorporating mindful practices won't guarantee a person has zero stress in their lifetime, it can improve the brain's capacity to view stressful situations with resiliency, optimism, and positivity, allowing a person to have a more stable mood and mindset in every activity they perform. Imagine the possibilities for yourself when you unlock the ability to better control your feelings and reactions.

This practice requires an openness that often becomes an obstacle for beginners. Many people have the best intentions for starting a practice of mindfulness through meditation but soon become bored or distracted, giving up quickly since they feel they're not performing the exercise correctly. If this sounds familiar, allow me to reassure you that staying with this practice over time does pay off exponentially. You can learn to stay mindful in everything you try, and with the help of techniques like meditation, deep breathing, and body scans, you can enrich every other activity or task that you set out to complete.

The Importance of Getting Grounded

Begin this journey by understanding that there are hundreds of techniques to assist you with mindfulness throughout your day, but you don't need to focus on every one of them to gain some initial benefits from a mindful practice. Incorporating even small mindful techniques for a short time can show positive and measurable benefits to the frontal and prefrontal regions of the brain, leading researchers to conclude that mindfulness practices positively reshape a brain's gray matter, prefrontal cortex, amygdala, and hippocampus (Hölzel et al., 2011).

The key to starting this, as with any new practice, is to not get overwhelmed from the beginning. It's time to get grounded in the process and not take on too much at once. While this book will offer many techniques and suggestions to help with mindfulness, it's important to choose what's right for you. You can rest assured that incorporating any techniques will help you feel more calm and confident throughout your day, but it's best to start first with those that will help you become grounded in a future practice of mindfulness so that you'll want to continue.

In the upcoming chapters, you'll find sections at the end that will offer mindful ideas that connect to the chapter topic. These are meant to give you an immediate way to put your learning into practice as you develop a more mindful approach to life.

Choose what you believe will work best for you based on your schedule and goals. While it's great to try new ideas, if you attempt a technique that feels uncomfortable for you, allow yourself to try something different while remaining open to learning and growing from the process.

Developing your skills in mindfulness does become easier with time and practice, but it will take patience on your part as well. The openness that you bring to these techniques will assist you in getting the most benefits from your practice.

Remember, first, to focus on small ways to improve and develop your practice each day.

Mindful Ideas for Getting Grounded

The following ideas are suggestions for grounding yourself in a practice full of new opportunities for you. These are simply ideas that can help an individual prepare for having a more mindful attitude. These are also ideas that will help to quickly soothe your mind when you're feeling stressed or anxious.

In future chapters, you'll learn more about specific meditation practices and techniques but, for now, allow these ideas to guide you in becoming more ready to grow an openness for your practice.

- Find a comfortable chair, close your eyes, and simply sit with your thoughts for five minutes.

- Create or find a space within your home that brings you a sense of calmness or happiness.

- Find a soft object that makes you feel satisfied or calm, like a blanket, pillow, or cozy pajamas.

- Buy, print, or draw a calendar to track mindfulness practices.

- Choose one hour within the next week. Reserve this time for a favorite activity that you complete alone such as having a bath or shower, taking a nap, or going for a walk.

- Start paying attention to the lighting in your home. Would you change anything? Is the lighting calming or not? What would you change (if anything)?

- Find blank paper or a blank notebook to begin journaling during your future mindfulness journey. Start setting a timer for 10 minutes each day and free-write during these minutes (in later chapters, I'll discuss topics that will help you focus).

- Make your bed (focus on making your sleeping space clean and cozy).

- Make a list of three people you can rely on. These could be considered your go-to friends or family members for times when you need help.

- Write a list of five songs (or musical artists) that you find calming or satisfying.

- Think about one outfit that makes you feel confident (wear it this week).

- Find a place in your home to sit and observe your surroundings without judging them for 10 minutes. What do you notice?

- Create one mantra for yourself. This could be as simple as "stay present." Say this mantra to yourself each morning as the first thing you do when you wake up.

- If anxious, take three slow deep breaths in and out (we'll build on breathing techniques in a later chapter).

- Take a short 15- or 20-minute walk today. Pay attention to your senses. What do you see, hear, and smell while walking?

- Count from 1 to 10 slowly, then count backward from 10 to 1 slowly.

- Find a candle or scent for your home that makes you feel calm. Close your eyes and smell this scent when you feel anxious.

- Gently tap up and down your arms with your fingertips for twenty seconds while breathing. Then, stop and relax. Notice how you feel.

- Complete a small task to feel a sense of accomplishment. This should be something you're good at and can finish with ease.

- Walk outside and simply breathe for five minutes.

- Sit in a chair or lie on your bed when you're anxious. Close your eyes and think of being in your favorite place, like a field of flowers or a spa.

- Delete an unnecessary app from your phone (start small; we'll continue a discussion of reducing phone use and distractions in future chapters).

- Keep your bedroom dark when sleeping (see bonus content about sleep in the appendix).

- Wash your hands and face (you'll be surprised at how grounding and satisfying this can feel).

- Talk to someone you admire and who exudes positivity.

- Take a break to read a book for 30 minutes to an hour.

- Move locations (from one room to another to gain a new perspective).

- Create a character for your feelings. For example, "Draw or describe [your anxiety] as a little gremlin puppet, an animal, or a cartoonish ghost. Then you can mentally narrate the story of your interactions with anxiety" (Regan, 2023). This can help you understand that your emotions don't have to control you and that you're in charge of your reactions to situations.

- Recognize yourself. Where are you in your life at this moment? State the time, month, and year aloud. Describe what you're doing today. This can help to bring your awareness to the present moment.

- Watch or listen to one of my free guided meditation practices (see appendix). Start noticing what you may learn to enjoy about the practice of meditation.

- Consider what you're grateful for today. Think of three items, people, or concepts that you could show gratitude for. Use your gratitude journal to complete this exercise or download one of these free templates to write your response.

Key Takeaways

- Communication takes place in the brain's message center, allowing us to receive and exchange information through synapses and the release of chemicals.

- The brain's plasticity changes and adapts to new experiences, whether positive or negative.

- Mindful techniques help calm and observe thoughts so that stress is alleviated and a growth mindset can form.

When you start to consider what options will help you feel the most grounded to create a more positive mindset, remember to start slowly and use positive self-talk. Any practice is difficult to begin without an open mind and a willingness to try something new, so offer yourself the chance to stay curious about your own exploration of mindfulness.

"Stay curious, stay open… and let's see what happens."

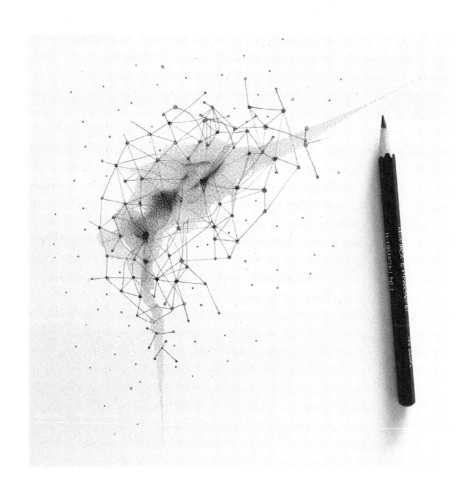

Chapter 2:

Mindfulness and the Brain

If you imagine the physical attributes of the human brain, what do you picture? You might visualize a scene from a science fiction movie where a wet, pinkish blob with wavy grooves floats in a jar or sits on a silver tray in a laboratory. Typically, the physical aspects of the brain don't appear to be much, but the functions of this mysterious organ are phenomenal.

Our brains are made up of tissue that constantly directs our responses, senses, movement, communication abilities, memory, feelings, language, and thinking (Maldonado & Alsayouri, 2023). When we feel excited, angry, overwhelmed, surprised, or fearful, our brain works hard to make sense of it all. Our brain naturally works to do this for us, but any damage to or disease of the brain can interrupt the signals and messages that are trying to move from one place to another. Studying the sections of the brain and their functions can help us better understand why self-care and preservation of our memory are significant to our well-being.

In this section, we'll examine the main parts of the brain and their functions so we can understand how they impact our mood and mindset. Because reinforcement and cognitive training have been proven to positively impact brain activity, it's helpful to know the major areas that are involved in brain function so we can understand how a practice of mindfulness can be beneficial.

What We Know About the Brain

Though the brain still contains many mysteries, scientific research has allowed us to have a deeper understanding of the brain's functions. The right and left sides of the brain, collectively called the cerebrum, contain folds and ridges at their surface (Maldonado & Alsayouri, 2023). The cerebrum connects to the brainstem and helps to control behaviors, feelings, memory, and motor and sensory functions (Maldonado & Alsayouri, 2023). The left side of the brain assists with language and processing logical concepts, while the right side controls more creative and intuitive ideas. The two sides work in tandem to make sense of the abstract ideas as well as the tangible concepts that we encounter each day.

The Four Lobes

Within these sections of the brain, four lobes help fine-tune even more of our processing skills (Maldonado & Alsayouri, 2023).

Frontal Lobe

This lobe takes charge of the language, cognitive, and motor functions allowing a person to regulate mood, self-awareness, and personality. Think of this area of the brain as the part that gives you the ability to plan and control what you want to do.

Parietal Lobe

The parietal lobe helps a person clarify sensory information and assists with memory. Without this part, we wouldn't be able to process temperatures on our skin or spatial awareness.

Temporal Lobe

The temporal lobe functions as a processing plant for language both written and spoken. This area lets us store and retrieve information so that we can recognize and hold memories from the past.

Occipital Lobe

Finally, the occipital lobe works to interpret visual. This lobe helps us with facial recognition and depth perception.

The Cerebellum

Next, the cerebellum is a center for controlling movements and motor functions. "The cerebellum also aids in various cognitive functions such as attention, language, pleasure response, and fear memory" (Maldonado & Alsayouri, 2023). It's in this area that our brain works to perfect how we want to move our bodies. "New studies are exploring the cerebellum's roles in thought, emotions, and social behavior, as well as its possible involvement in addiction, autism, and schizophrenia" (Johns Hopkins Medicine, 2022).

The Brainstem

Finally, the brainstem consists of the midbrain, pons, and medulla, which are areas that work together to control bodily functions. The brainstem connects the cerebrum to the spinal cord and makes connections to control the "autonomic functions such as breathing, temperature regulation, respiration, heart rate, wake-sleep cycles, coughing, sneezing, digestion, vomiting, and swallowing" (Maldonado & Alsayouri, 2023).

How Mindful Practices Can Shape the Brain

Each day, our brain works hard to make sense of our surroundings and to send messages to the parts of our bodies that we want to function properly. While the brain does this with minimal realized effort, it's actually working quite hard to learn lessons and categorize events. As our brain retains information from each experience, it adds to the rewiring that occurs as a result.

When an individual is placed in a situation that calls for a reaction, their brain works to choose a response that will best protect that individual.

You've most likely heard about the idea of "fight" or "flight," but these reactions cause our brains and bodies to hang on to the memories of these responses each time they occur so that we can learn from the experience. The way we respond to circumstances impacts the gray matter, or the tissue in our brains that allows us to function and make intelligent decisions (Hölzel et al., 2011). The brain sends messages through hormone secretions of cortisol and adrenaline, providing a person with a response that protects them in many cases, but one that also adds to their mental and physical stress over time.

If you've ever noticed tense shoulder muscles or a clenched jaw at the end of a stressful workday, you can understand the impact that experiences can physically have on the body. Over time, the body and mind continue holding onto this stress if they don't have an outlet for a release from the tension. Heart disease, depression, anxiety, Alzheimer's disease, obesity, and gastrointestinal issues are just some of the health risks associated with long-term stress (R. Morgan Griffin, 2010).

In a fast-paced world inundated with distractions, nurturing our brain health has never been more crucial. Amidst the chaos, mindfulness emerges as a powerful tool. Through deliberate attention to the present moment, mindfulness invites us to observe our thoughts, emotions, and sensations without judgment. In doing so, we can foster a deeper understanding of the intricate workings of our minds.

Research increasingly demonstrates the myriad benefits of mindfulness for brain health, from reducing stress and anxiety to enhancing cognitive function and emotional regulation. Some recent findings have focused on how a long-term daily practice of mindful meditation can increase grey matter density. Grey matter is the part of the brain and spinal cord primarily composed of neuronal cell bodies and dendrites, essential for processing information and carrying out cognitive functions. It impacts our emotions, communication, and decision-making abilities. Mindful meditation has also been linked to helping thicken the hippocampus, which is associated with emotional regulation and memory.

Regular Mindfulness

To settle our minds and bodies, our brain requires activities that offer a break from the typical and give us a chance to recalibrate our physical and mental well-being. Many believe that the practice of mindfulness must solely focus on meditation, but there are numerous ways to both soothe and refresh a mind and body.

When a person incorporates mindful practices into their day, they're likely to feel a sense of calmness, gratitude, and hope that, over time, helps them build an intimate connection to their place in the world and feel happier and more satisfied with themselves overall.

To demonstrate how mindful practices offer a sense of connection even if practiced alone, imagine the way you feel when you've had a chance to participate in an activity that you love versus one that you don't. How do you feel when the activity is done? When finished with something you don't like doing, you may feel a sense of relief that the work is done, but you may also feel tired and unable to complete other tasks afterward.

Mindful activities offer us a chance to spend moments interacting with our thoughts and feelings and focusing on something in a calm manner so that we then can absorb the energy this offers us and use it to perform other activities mindfully.

Though staying mindful is not magic, it offers beneficial assets for overall living, including a new awareness and openness to experiences and people, greater empathy and compassion for others, and the ability to understand stress and respond to it with a regulated approach.

In one study of the impact that mindfulness can offer, researchers studied the brains of individuals who had meditated for approximately 30 minutes a day for eight weeks consecutively (Hölzel et al., 2011). When measuring brain activity, these researchers found that the gray matter of participants' brains had become more concentrated than at the start of their experiment, demonstrating that the areas that trigger memories, a sense of self, and empathy were more fully engaged over time as a result of their mindful practice. Research has also shown that the longer someone practices meditation, the better their concentration and attention (Baron Short et al, 2010).

In my own research, preliminary studies using functional magnetic resonance imaging (fMRI), which is a way to show brain network connections, have shown the potential for mindfulness practices to change brain networks in the context of neurological conditions (Wong et al, 2024).

While mysteries of the brain are still getting unlocked by researchers daily, it's helpful to have some insight into which practices and techniques can provide mindful benefits to a person.

In our bustling, non-stop world, mindfulness can feel like a distant luxury. Yet, as William Henry Davies poetically mused, "What is this life if, full of care, We have no time to stand and stare?"

The constant flux of our modern lives makes mindfulness not only challenging but also increasingly essential.

At its core, mindfulness invites us to embrace the present moment fully, acknowledging our thoughts, emotions, and sensations as they arise in response to the world around us. By cultivating this awareness, we can alleviate unnecessary worries, savor life's joys, and gain deeper insights into ourselves.

While integrating mindfulness into our daily routines is invaluable, setting aside dedicated time for mindfulness practices can amplify its benefits. Here are various techniques you can incorporate into your day:

- Mindfulness Meditation: During life's hustle, whether on a crowded subway or halted at a red light, dedicate a moment to focus on your breath. Simply observe its ebb and flow, allowing its rhythm to serve as an anchor to the present moment, grounding you amidst the chaos. You could also schedule this into your home routine, for example by setting aside ten minutes in the evening as you wind down at the end of a busy day.

- Open Awareness: Engage your senses fully, immersing yourself in the rich tapestry of the world around you. Take note of the sounds, colors, and sensations that surround you. This practice cultivates a deep connection to the present moment, fostering a sense of presence.

- Body Scan: Set aside a moment to tune into your body, scanning for any areas of tension, discomfort, or subtle sensations. Without passing judgment, simply acknowledge what you feel, embracing the unity of your physical and emotional selves. This practice bridges the gap between mind and body, fostering a sense of wholeness and self-awareness.

- Mindful Movement: Embrace movement with yoga, tai chi or pilates. With each stretch and extension, hone in on the rhythm of your breath and the sensations through your body. Transform each movement into an opportunity for mindful awareness, grounding yourself in the present moment.

- 3-Step Breathing Spaces: The 3-Step Breathing Spaces is a technique taught in Mindfulness-Based Cognitive Therapy (MBCT). It starts with open awareness, taking a minute to notice what is present in the moment with your emotions, sensations within your body, your thought patterns or concerns. Next, gather your attention and anchor it on your breath, for approximately a minute. Take deep, intentional breaths, allowing each inhalation and exhalation to anchor you firmly in the present moment. Pause briefly between each breath and find sanctuary amidst the chaos, nurturing a sense of peace and tranquillity within. Finally, expand your awareness from your breath to your whole body. Notice how you feel now compared to when you started.

- Mindfulness of Thoughts and Emotions: Delve into the depths of your inner landscape, cultivating a keen awareness of your thoughts and emotions as they surface. Observe them with gentle curiosity, allowing them to arise and pass without clinging or judgment. In this practice of radical acceptance, embrace the full spectrum of your human experience, fostering a sense of self-understanding.

We'll expand on some of these techniques in the following chapters and show how these practices can support different aspects of your life and brain health. See the appendix for audioguides introducing the above practices.

Mindful Ideas to Enhance Brain Health

Practicing mindful meditation, which we'll discuss in a later chapter, can help the mind and body reset.

Meanwhile, the following ideas offer a way to supplement your day with brief, achievable self-care practices and activities to keep your brain active and alert. The ideas outlined here are ones to consider if you're looking to calm stress responses in your body and gain an improved sense of emotional regulation and awareness over time.

As a reminder, the ideas that follow are not meant to be completed all at once. They're not even meant to be tackled as a set. Instead, this list offers you a menu of options to choose from if you'd like to try an activity that nurtures brain health.

- Set intentional limits on screen time and practice mindful technology use by taking breaks to rest your eyes and refocus your attention away from digital distractions.

- Simplify decision-making by reducing the number of options whenever feasible, as an abundance of choices can overwhelm the mind and lead to mental fatigue.

- Make to-do lists and cross items off. Notice how the sense of accomplishment feels.

- Find opportunities to create routines each day. For example, start by going to bed and waking up around the same time each day. Keep a diary to track how this makes you feel throughout the day.

- Protect your time and create boundaries for yourself. Notice how you feel after giving yourself some time to rest and recharge.

- Make a list of the top three people who bring you happiness and send them a message to tell them how thankful you are to have them in your life.

- Make a list of the top three things that bring you peace. Schedule dedicated time in your week to them. Whether its coffee in a café, seeing a friend, walking your dog or having a lazy day.

- Find ways to reward yourself for a job well done or for accomplishing tasks. Let this reward motivate your brain to keep achieving.

- Keep a gratitude journal. At the end of each day, spend a little time reflecting on your day and write down three things you're grateful for. They can be as small as a delicious snack you had or a kind remark from a loved one.

- Practice active listening during conversations, meetings, or when enjoying music, fully engaging your senses and reducing mental distractions.

- What is something you've always wanted to know more about? Give yourself time to explore your curiosity, whether by reading a book, watching a documentary, attending a talk or visiting a museum.

- Spend time in nature. Green spaces (like a park, forest or field) and blue spaces (like the ocean, a lake or river) are proven to help soothe our minds and promote feelings of contentment.

- Eat foods that are rich in vitamins and antioxidants, such as spinach, kale, omega-3 fatty acids, olive oil, and avocado. Limit overeating by moderating portion sizes.

- Stay connected with your community and consider participating in social activities.

- Learn tai chi, a gentle form of martial arts, to improve balance, coordination, and cognitive function while promoting relaxation.

- Play brain games such as puzzles and notice how it feels to give yourself a challenge.

- Limit your alcohol intake. You could keep a diary of when you drink alcohol and how it makes you feel. Monitor how it impacts you and make changes that support how you want to feel.

- Schedule regular check-ups with physicians for things like eye checks and with your dentist. These small things can feel very gratifying and provide you with a sense that you're looking after yourself proactively.

- Embrace the journey to quit smoking as a mindful practice, cultivating awareness of the harmful effects of smoking on both physical health and mental well-being.

- Limit sugar in your diet, but don't force yourself to quit if you have a sweet tooth. Whenever you do eat something sweet, take your time, savor it and enjoy the moment.

- Set an alarm one hour before bedtime to remind your brain and body to start winding down for the night. Create a supportive routine for a restful night that includes stretching, journaling, a herbal tea, reading or anything else that helps.

NB: The above self-care ideas help settle your brain and body for regular mindfulness meditation practices. See Appendix for free audioguides on mindfulness meditations. Use these audioguides alongside the above self-care practices, as you embark on your "Year of Mindfulness".

Key Takeaways

When considering how to incorporate more mindful practices into your life, get creative with the opportunities that you're offered. Listen to your inner voice when deciding what activities feel right and worthwhile for you.

- Tissue in the brain controls sensory functions, movement, memory, and language.

- The four lobes of the brain—frontal, parietal, temporal, and occipital—allow a person to absorb, process, and react to experiences.

- The brainstem and cerebellum control certain movements of the body.

- Research studies show that the brain's gray matter and brain networks respond to mindful practices, with a positive impact on individuals.

As we move beyond our basic discussion of the ways that mindful practices impact the brain, we'll start examining more specific aspects of memory and cognitive functions for benefiting brain health.

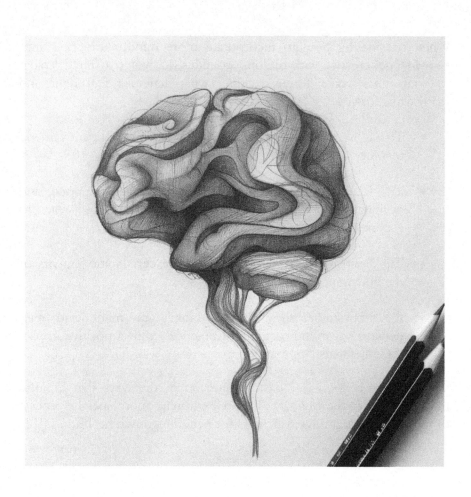

Chapter 3:

Memory and Mindfulness

Take a deep breath in, then a long breath out. What do you smell at this very moment? If you happen to be near a flower arrangement, air freshener, or certain food, you're likely to have an easier time quickly identifying what memory this particular scent might trigger for you.

The sense of smell is one of our most powerful senses that aids in memory. "The most distinctive characteristic of odor-evoked memories, however, and why they are important to human health and well-being is that they evoke more emotional and evocative recollections than memories triggered by any other cue" (Herz, 2016). You've probably had a memory that's been provoked by a particular sense in your recent past. For example, I can still remember the scent of fragrant oils in my grandmother's house and, when I smell a similar scent today, I'm transported right back to my visits to her house in my childhood.

We each have memories that are significant to us and ones that have helped shape our personalities. We are a species that learns through experience, and each memory we hold adds to our decision-making ability in the present. Therefore, our potential to tap into our mind's deep-rooted thoughts can offer clues about the kind of person we are, as well as what we strive to be.

The Power of the Mind and Memory

The conscious mind is dynamic and prolific. It works automatically without a person having to focus on the communication between synapses inside the brain. If you've ever experienced waking up in a location that's fairly unfamiliar to you, such as a friend's home or a hotel room, you've experienced your mind working quickly to recall your setting and make sense of your surroundings. Our conscious mind grabs onto and stores prior experiences and knowledge so that we remain familiar with situations that might otherwise feel uncomfortable.

So, what happens when an injury to the brain or a disease clouds the awareness of our surroundings or causes a lapse in memory? When this takes place, a person's cognitive skills and awareness may be impacted to the point where it's harder to focus and requires more time to process sensory information. An injury or disease affecting the brain can not only impact memory, but may also affect decision-making, multi-tasking abilities, and communication through speech or writing (Mayo Clinic, 2021). In addition, physical and behavioral changes may occur. In cases, for example, where a person experiences a head injury causing a concussion, blind spots, balance problems, mood swings, and difficulty in following along with a conversation have resulted (Mayo Clinic, 2021). When we consider the impact that the brain's basic functions have on everyday productivity, recollection, and language, any negative impact caused by head trauma can damage the brain's functionality.

Working and Episodic Memory

A person's ability to give their attention to a task and remember how to perform this task is vital to how we complete work, take care of ourselves, and interact with others daily. Working memory is a type of memory that holds short-term information so that we can effectively complete a task. Working to maintain our memory's potential or even to improve it has become an industry in our society, which highly values strategic ways of self-improvement and being productive. Learning how mindfulness can benefit the brain and memory can allow any individual to enhance the way they use their mental strengths throughout the day.

Episodic memory is a form of long-term memory, giving us the ability to recall specific events from the past. It guides our behavior and provides us with the capacity to make current and future decisions. Episodic memory is subject to both neurological insult and age-related decline (Brown et al., 2016). Intervening with protective practices like mindfulness training exercises may enhance a person's ability to preserve their episodic memory and recall events.

Mindfulness training comes in two main forms, "focused attention" and "open monitoring" (Brown et al., 2016). Focused attention training, or FA training, involves practical exercises that direct a person's attention and help them perceive their surroundings. This kind of mindfulness training has proven successful in helping individuals with tasks that require concentration and sustained focus. By practicing mindfulness training, the working memory becomes stronger and less likely to break down (Brown et al., 2016).

Mental Noting

Because memories from our past can trigger our sensory functions, it's no wonder that mindful practices can directly connect to the ability to improve memory. Practices such as yoga, meditation, and body scanning can assist in reminding us of certain events, but can also give us a chance to examine these events, with a calm and objective focus.

One popular technique to use during meditation is the process of "mental noting," in which a person acknowledges the thoughts they're having during meditation but allows these ideas to pass through the mind as if they're simply being observed by the participant (Kabat-Zinn, 1994). Some individuals imagine their thoughts floating in clouds or passing by them on written notes while mental noting occurs.

To try this mental noting for yourself, find a comfortable seat where you won't be interrupted for the next five minutes. Close your eyes and start breathing in and out slowly through your nose. At first, focus on calming your body and mind so that your brain has a chance to adjust to this practice. After a minute or two, you'll probably notice yourself having thoughts about what to do next, what your day has been like so far, what you want to eat for dinner, and so on.

This busy brain activity happens to everyone, especially those new to meditation, so don't allow yourself to feel frustrated by it. Instead, simply place the image or wording of your thought onto a cloud and picture it floating past you.

The purpose of this is to allow the thoughts in your busy mind the chance to be seen but not given power. With your eyes closed, you can visualize that they exist, but you can also learn to send them floating past you.

This experience takes some practice to feel comfortable with since, for many of us, we want to fixate on or accomplish a task when we first think of it. Don't worry—mental noting becomes easier with time.

As you practice this technique, consider the end goal as well. The process of practicing mental noting will allow you to sit and relax, observe your thoughts, and feel a calmness about each thought as you won't need to stress about accomplishing it within that exact moment. You simply learn to observe it, leave it, and deal with it when the time is right.

Brain Training for Memory

When was the last time you walked into a room and couldn't remember what you were there to do? Our brain is like a muscle, and when we work it, it gains strength. If you start thinking about your brain this way, it can help you make more positive choices about what activities you allow your brain to partake in and what you might need to stay away from.

While life presents us with stress and there's only so much a person can avoid, we do have some control over what we allow our bodies and minds to encounter daily. For example, getting poor sleep night after night can impact your mood and your ability to recall memories. While most people don't set out to get a poor night of sleep, they also may not do themselves any favors by watching television while they fall asleep or drinking caffeine too close to bedtime.

Just as a person might invest in a gym membership to feel healthier and build strength, practicing brain-training exercises can enhance memory over time and help the brain limit overstimulation. Like building muscle mass with repetition, focusing on repeated exercises for the brain can build the habit of strengthening memory.

Mindful techniques can help with brain training by allowing a person to focus more intently on their surroundings and pay closer attention to a task. One study of mindfulness found that training the brain to meditate or participate in mindful activities, like yoga, had a positive impact on episodic memory and gave individuals more motivation to complete activities beyond meditation and yoga (Brown et al., 2016). Think of brain training as the extra credit that improves your life. Incorporating brain training techniques can help maintain a sharper mind and prolong your brain's ability.

Mindful Ideas for Memory

To set yourself up for success with brain training, start by scheduling time for yourself so that you can create the mental and physical space you need. It's possible to complete brain training activities both at work and at home, but you'll need to start small to build endurance. Focus on completing small practices at first until your mind builds the habit of incorporating brain training into your day.

Just as with any activity, if you go at it too hard, you're likely to give up quickly, so take short moments to try one activity from the list below to start. You might want to try simply reserving ten minutes before bedtime to journal about your day or settle your brain with a guided meditation. Eventually, you can build to activities that require more brain power but, for now, start with something that will be easy for you to complete and will give your mind a quick sense of accomplishment.

The following ideas can help start you on your path toward getting more creative with your time and accomplishments. These ideas are general ways to take care of your brain. They can provide you with a starting point in adjusting your mindset to value the importance of brain health.

- Start the day by listing the top three things you need to accomplish.

- Take a 'screen break' every hour (walk around for several minutes before returning to a screen). Try stretching and pay attention to your body before you sit back down.

- Write a story of one memory from your childhood. Think about all the senses as you write: what can you see, hear, smell and taste? Discuss one of your childhood memories with your parents or another family member to see what they remember and compare your stories.

- Visit a library. Check out a new book that looks interesting to you and try reading for at least 30 minutes each day until you finish this book.

- Get seven to nine hours of consistent sleep each night (our brain thrives when we get the right amount of sleep for our body).

- Start writing down your dreams each morning. Do you notice any themes or messages that keep coming up? How might they relate to your day-to-day?

- Explore your curiosity and learn something new about a topic you've been interested in for a while. Visit a museum or workshop, attend a talk, or read a book about the topic.

- Visualize your day or an important event before it happens. Walk your brain through each detail before it happens.

- Host a games night with friends and/or family. Plan some fun activities to do together, such as a board game, charades or perhaps a quiz.

- Read a biography of someone you admire or know little about.

- Write a journal entry reflecting on all the events you remember from your day.

- Try out a new physical hobby that requires you to learn a sequence, such as a dance class. Support your memory by attending each week and building on the steps you learn.

- Mix things up in your routine to grow your memory of the places you attend regularly. You could take a new route to work, walk instead of driving or catching public transport, visit a new café on the weekend – these all help to engage different parts of your brain and memory.

- Challenge yourself with language in new ways. You could learn a new language, learn basic sign language through a class or read up about new words and vocabulary to use in your daily life.

- Write a journal entry about one conversation you had during the day. What details can you remember?

- Teach someone a skill or something you know about. Teaching others is a great way to consolidate our knowledge and memory of the things we are interested in and care about.

- Spend time with people you love to create meaningful memories!

NB: The above self-care ideas help settle your brain and body for regular mindfulness meditation practices. See Appendix for free audioguides on mindfulness meditations. Use these audioguides alongside the above self-care practices, as you embark on your "Year of Mindfulness".

Key Takeaways

By now, you've probably considered how the mindful ideas within these chapters can be added to your life. Some are easier activities than others, so choose ones that you believe will add value to your practice of mindfulness.

- Cognitive abilities and awareness are impacted when the brain suffers injuries, impacting awareness, memory, and communication.

- Training the brain with mindfulness exercises can improve memory and recall functions of the brain.

- Communication within the brain becomes more challenging with unconsciousness.

- Activities such as mental noting can lead to an observation of thoughts without judgment.

- Self-awareness and memory improve with mindful techniques that let individuals focus on their present situation.

In addition to aiding memory, mindful activities benefit a brain's cognitive functioning. In the next chapter, we'll look closer at the ways that emotional intelligence can improve through mindful life choices and practices.

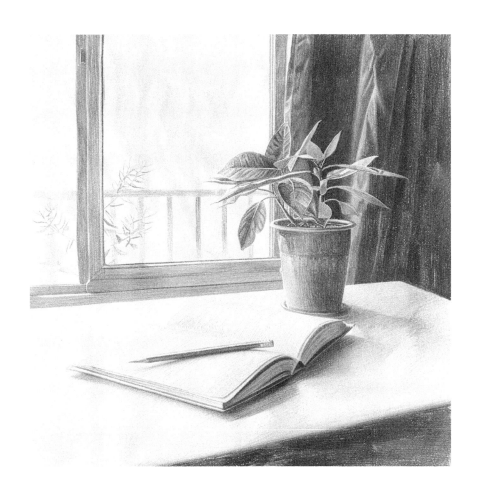

Chapter 4:

Increasing Cognitive Functioning

Through Mindful Techniques

You've heard it before, but the idea of "never stop learning" truly matters when it comes to improving the functions of the brain. While you've already learned about the importance that brain training can have on memory, it's now time to take a closer look at how mindful techniques nurture the brain's other significant functions. Not only does this build brain strength through cognitive activities, but it also offers a way to calm emotions and center one's thoughts on the present.

Imagine you're just waking up in the morning and you have thoughts of your various to-do lists running through your mind. You quickly go about your typical morning routine, brushing your teeth, showering, getting dressed, and eating breakfast, while the ominous reminders of what you need to accomplish hover over you, making each task less enjoyable.

Now, picture yourself having the ability to wake up and complete the same morning chores, but feeling calm and composed while you focus on each task and staying in the moment as you complete it.

If this sounds impossible or impractical, consider for a moment why your brain is locked into trying to multi-task each day. For many of us, our thoughts tend to race when our bodies are on autopilot, doing the repetitive activities that we've trained them to do over the years. To some degree, our minds have grown "bored" with the physical tasks that we've performed over and over and are seeking ways to utilize our time more efficiently. Despite what we tell ourselves, multitasking tends to turn out poorly for many of us.

If this feels relatable, the practice of mindfulness can help you grow and adapt to change. By adding mindful practices into your day and training your brain to have a designated time to concentrate on the present moment, you can build a habit that supports your ability to focus throughout your day. For example, meditating is one way to center the mind and observe thoughts as they float in and out of our brain, but most of us wouldn't attempt to ride a stationary bike, watch a movie, and make a sandwich while trying to meditate, right?

Settling into a practice of meditation requires us to set aside other tasks for the day and feel stillness for a designated time. This is often what turns some people off about practicing meditation, as well. We're so busy completing activities throughout the day that we might feel it's a waste of time to pause for a meditation break. This is often the mindset that holds individuals back from unlocking the benefits of this practice.

Instead of viewing a mindful practice as an interruption, think of it as a way to incorporate mindfulness into any daily task. While brushing our teeth, eating a meal, or washing dishes, we can stay mindful and aware of our thoughts and feel gratitude that we can participate in such activities.

Boosting the Brain

To gain the rewards of a mindful practice, we might first need to understand just what exactly we're getting ourselves into. Mindfulness is a practice that's rooted in many worldviews and religions, from Hinduism to Buddhism to Christianity.

As a practice, it became more widely known in the Western world when author, professor, and creator of the "Stress Reduction Clinic," Jon Kabat-Zinn, began teaching others about the value of mindfulness in conjunction with stress reduction (Kabat-Zinn, 2013). It was a revolutionary approach, when he first introduced this philosophy as a treatment for chronic pain. On a personal note, watching a documentary about Jon Kabat-Zinn's work had inspired me to bring mindfulness research into the neurological context.

This philosophy emphasizes mindfulness as a non-judgmental approach to our thoughts so we can train the mind to acknowledge internal and external experiences. Doing so gives us a chance to realize our ideas without the emotions or pressure that we tend to place on them.

Think of your brain as a source of energy. When we stimulate it with new, varied information, it's brought to life and gains vitality. In the same vein, when we train it through the repetition of mindful activities that feel comfortable, it learns to rely on this source of nurturing.

Holistic Yoga

Since incorporating a holistic yoga practice will work to invigorate the mind, body, and spirit, this activity can be the perfect way to begin your journey of mindfulness. In studies on well-being and resilience among various populations, researchers found that "even a single yoga class had a statistically significant effect on improving mood among 113 psychiatric inpatients. Patients were significantly less tense/anxious, less depressed/dejected, less angry/hostile, less confused/bewildered, and less fatigued after participating in a yoga class" (Hartfiel et al., 2011).

Holistic yoga is meant to care for the human as a whole, and this practice encourages a person to participate in movement that feels right for their body and mind. The purpose is to gain self-awareness and slow our thoughts down so we can exist in a state of present awareness. Therefore, the practice of accepting what a body is capable of and adapting movements for that capability is encouraged. Holistic yoga also focuses on breath awareness that will support a calm consciousness and emphasizes the harmony of the body as a whole through healthy lifestyle choices.

Mindful Meditation

By more fully engaging the mind's senses and attention, an individual can gain mental openness and awareness that translate to numerous activities in life. Practicing meditation that focuses on mindful observations of thoughts and feelings can greatly influence how we can relieve stress and strengthen our mental capabilities. "Studies using self-report data from healthy individuals have shown that mindfulness meditation decreased negative mood states, improved positive mood states, and reduced distractive and ruminative thoughts and behaviors" (Hölzel, Lazar, et al., 2011).

A variety of mindful meditation practice techniques exist. As you start out in your mindfulness journey it can be helpful to choose a practice that feels comforting as well as engaging. This way, you're more likely to stick with a long-term practice to receive even more benefits from the incorporation of mindfulness. While mindful meditation takes some effort, its benefit is that it's a free and straightforward way to feel a sense of relief as you notice your thoughts without letting your mind remain absorbed in them.

If you'd like to practice mindfully meditating, now is as good a time as any to give it a try. See the appendix for access to free audioguides to assist you with this. To get a small taste of the bonus content available there, let's try a quick practice now.

Sit in a quiet location where you won't be interrupted for the next few minutes. Set a timer for yourself if needed, but try not to watch the seconds tick by as you meditate. The timer is simply there to bring you back to the present moment when you're finished meditating. Now, close your eyes and breathe. Notice how you feel in both your mind and body. Focus on your breathing. After several minutes you may notice that your mind has wandered to other thoughts. This is quite normal and expected. When this happens, gently bring your thoughts back to your breathing. As ideas come into your mind, you could place them in an imaginary box or on a cloud and visualize them passing by you. Simply observe, without becoming caught up in the thoughts or feel stressed about them, and watch them as they drift away.

After meditating for any amount of time, it's important to gently guide yourself into the next activity. Give yourself a few minutes to absorb the effects of the practice you just completed, and then move mindfully on to your next task.

Additional Meditation Techniques

Other meditative practices are a subset of mindful meditation and emphasize mind-body awareness, compassion, and focused attention. These practices have been therapeutic in helping patients and participants relieve pain and anxious thoughts.

Mind-Body Awareness

Having a conscious awareness of the way one's body feels and reacts to its surroundings brings an awareness that can help an individual slow down and take note of the way the brain and body work in unison.

In a study of the effects of mind-body meditation practices, 32 breast cancer survivors focused on relaxing parts of their bodies during meditation to recognize what areas felt tense or uncomfortable (Valluri et al., 2024). In doing so, participants were able to understand that their tension was connected to memories of the trauma they experienced from their illness. They were able to use this knowledge to bring more positive thoughts to the areas of their bodies that needed attention and relaxation.

Compassion

Because meditative practices hold foundational ties to Buddhism, ideas of self-love and kindness have always been part of the practice. The concept of having enough compassion for oneself to observe a thought judgment-free allows an individual to create a positive connection between mind and body. We can have an awareness of our strengths and weaknesses and use this to better understand the choices we make and the results they have.

In a study of loving-kindness practices, veterans who had faced traumatic experiences and had a history of anger engaged in meditation that focused on compassion (Valluri et al., 2024). They focused on deep-breathing practices as well as self-compassion and found that stressful thinking subsided with this technique.

Focused Attention

There are a few ways to practice focused attention.

If you've ever given yourself a pep talk before a stressful event or have repeated a positive affirmation to yourself, you've practiced something similar to focused attention meditation. By honing in on a positive aspect of a situation, the idea is that an individual can decrease their anxious thoughts or physical pain.

Transcendental Meditation (TM), participants have effectively reduced tension by focusing on a word or phrase, like repeating a mantra (Valluri et al., 2024). This allows them to bring forth a positive focus and reduce stressful thoughts.

Mindfulness-based cognitive therapy (MBCT) also offers a practical approach to managing our attention. By combining elements of mindfulness meditation with principles of cognitive therapy, MBCT helps individuals cultivate awareness of the present moment. Through gentle exercises, MBCT encourages us to observe our thoughts and feelings without judgment, allowing us to disengage from automatic reactions and choose where to direct our attention.

Focused Attention practices could even be just sitting in silence, e.g. for 10 minutes, and following our breath.

Over time, these practices strengthen our ability to focus, enhancing our concentration and clarity in daily life. Whether it's at work, in relationships, or during moments of solitude, mindfulness equips us with valuable tools to navigate the challenges of modern life with greater ease and presence.

Emotional Intelligence

Do you know someone who seems to have a high IQ but has difficulty keeping their emotional state regulated, or has setbacks when it comes to adaptability? We've now reached a topic that, for many, is hard to recognize and even harder to gain a desire to change since the qualities of emotional intelligence tend to be more vague than other more measurable forms of intelligence.

Emotional intelligence uses an internal awareness to allow us to take control of emotions and positively guide thoughts so we can feel satisfied and less stressed (Jiménez-Picón et al., 2021). This type of intelligence provides us with the ability to communicate productively and proactively. It also lets us deal effectively with any stressors or conflicts in a practical manner.

Think of emotional intelligence as a helpful, confident inner voice that leads us to a greater awareness of ourselves and our relationships with others. Its four attributes—self-management, self-awareness, social awareness, and relationship management—play an integral role in our ability to feel empathetic, clear-minded, and adaptable (Segal et al., 2023). Using mindful meditation, individuals can bring awareness and attention to the aspects that improve emotional intelligence traits. Incorporating a practice of mindful meditation can help those struggling to connect with the qualities of emotional intelligence, giving them an outlet for reducing their stress and gaining self-positivity.

Mindful Ideas for Alertness and Emotional Intelligence

The practice of mindfulness roots itself in the idea that an individual can cultivate self-awareness to assist them in relationships with others. It's important to think of ways to communicate effectively with others and understand that self-improvement is possible.

The following mindful ideas can provide a sense of focus while reminding individuals that they can learn to manage their feelings and emotions each day. Some of these suggestions are thoughts to ponder or write about, and some are techniques to put into practice.

Remember to make these activities your own by adapting them to your lifestyle.

- Reflect on how your emotions or feelings impact your day. Do you notice any that are too strong, not enough, or just right?

- Think of a recent conflict you had with another person. Without becoming angry or emotional, how would you prevent or resolve this conflict if you could experience it again?

- Tap into your empathetic self. Walk yourself through a scenario from another person's perspective.

- Practice active listening skills. As you talk with another person, engage in the conversation fully, paraphrase what they say, and use non-verbal cues.

- Celebrate one positive accomplishment (even small ones!) at the end of each day.

- When you're feeling stressed, practice deep breathing. Breathe in through your nose slowly for 30 seconds and then gently release the breath through your mouth. Try three deep breaths before making any quick decisions.

- Consider the people or ideas that might trigger you throughout the day and reflect on proactive ways to address them. It might mean rethinking some boundaries or having honest conversations about whether certain people are adding value in your life. Remember to breathe deeply as you consider this.

- Trust yourself and your intuition. Know that your ideas matter and have value.

- Start to trust others and see the best in them (this will help them trust you more in return). One small way to do this is to ask for help when you need it and trust that the person you ask can support you proactively.

- Realize that your reactions to conversations and situations are a choice (you control these).

- Create personal, achievable goals for yourself.

- If you have the means and ability, plan some travel to experience a new place or culture. Remember, you don't need to go far to achieve this. You could even try to visit a new or familiar part of your town and pretend you're a tourist – what might you see or discover with this perspective?

- Think about social activities, hobbies or sports you used to love that you haven't made time for recently. Reach out and get started again.

- Ask questions. This will not only show others you're interested in their ideas and advice, but you'll also learn answers and make discoveries about them.

- Be okay with the unknown and try not to become overwhelmed by things you can't have definitive answers to.

- Reflect on how much of what you say or think is actually a complaint. Make a diary to keep track of this. How could you reframe these thoughts in a positive way instead? Can you change the complaint? If not, how might you let it go for good?

- Stay present (meditating helps with this). Avoid ruminating too much on past experiences if these no longer serve you.

- Try doing something nice for someone (take a meal to their house, donate clothes to a charity, sweep someone's driveway, etc.)

- Listen to conversations happening around you (without eavesdropping). Pay attention to how others interact and listen to one another.

- Motivate yourself (listen to music that pumps you up, get a pep talk from a positive person, be a person you'd want to be friends with, etc.).

- Practice ignoring your phone (put it in a drawer while you work or exercise if needed).

- Sit and drink herbal tea as you clear your mind and recharge your energy for the day. Try my free audio meditation "A Mindful Cup of Tea."(see appendix)

- Stick to a schedule. When it's time to leave work, have something to look forward to afterward.

- Hold yourself accountable. Check in with your emotions throughout the day and notice what you're feeling.

- Start (or complete!) a craft project.

- Enter experiences with an open mind as if you can learn and grow from the process.

NB: *The above self-care ideas help settle your brain and body for regular mindfulness meditation practices. See Appendix for free audioguides on mindfulness meditations. Use these audioguides alongside the above self-care practices, as you embark on your "Year of Mindfulness".*

Key Takeaways

Each time you're able to gain awareness about your feelings, body, or mind, you'll be one step closer to having a stronger relationship with yourself and appreciating your energy and positivity. This will naturally benefit those around you as your gratitude transfers to them, as well.

- Incorporate mindful practices into a daily routine and start training the mind to focus on the present moment. This can help develop a habit that enhances overall focus.

- Mindful practices should help remove judgment from thoughts so the mind can acknowledge internal and external experiences.

Activities like holistic yoga and mindful meditation give a person a chance to experiment with this idea.

- Mind-body awareness, compassion, and focused attention help relieve pain and stressful thoughts.

- A person can improve emotional intelligence traits through mindful meditation and bring awareness to their emotions.

In understanding how we can begin incorporating techniques that will help us to stay more mindful before, during, and after activities such as yoga and meditation, it's important to stay clear about why we're adding this to our lives. Mindfulness allows us to gain more control of our emotional and physical world by giving us a new perspective.

To reiterate the benefits of this practice, we'll next take a look at the impact that stressful circumstances can have on our well-being so that we can better understand the importance of dedicating our time to mindful activities.

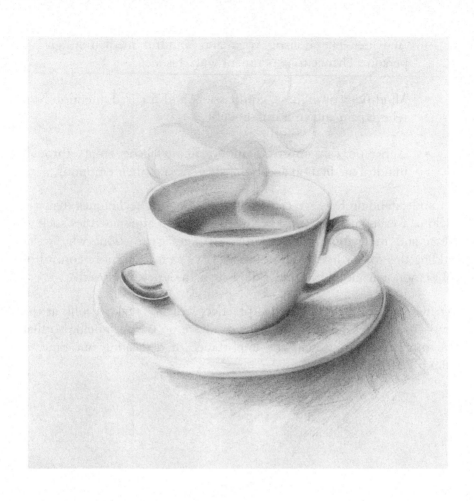

Chapter 5:

Understanding Stress—A Mindful

Approach

You awake on a rainy Monday morning, still groggy from staying up too late the night before because you wanted to finish the movie you were watching. What was it again? You're now having difficulty even remembering. You roll over in bed and blink your eyes a few times to take a strained look at the clock. You see the numbers 7:00 as your eyes start to feel heavy and close again. Wait! 7 a.m.!

You jump out of bed in a panic and look around the room. You see your suitcase packed and clothes laid out, but even if you leave now, you'll never make it in time to catch your 8 a.m. flight to your work conference. You speed around the room, wondering why you stayed up so late, why you forgot to set your alarm for an earlier time, and, in general, why you can't seem to get anything right.

As you throw your clothes on, grab your bags, and complete the world's fastest toothbrushing session, your shoulders and neck tighten. Once you're out the door and in your car, you feel a glimmer of hope that you can make it to the gate and shout for the staff to keep the doors open for just one more minute. You look at the clock in the car. 7:20 a.m. How will you get through security and run fast enough to make it on time? You then notice the cars in front of you slowing down. Ah! Traffic! No, this can't be happening!

By the time you've waited behind a line of cars for what feels like forever, your mind starts racing with the "what ifs." *What if I forgot to lock the front door? What if I can't eat anything until I get to my hotel and I'm starving on the plane? What if my presentation at the conference goes terribly? Oh, no! My presentation!* You glance at the back seat of your car where your suitcase is resting comfortably—but your laptop is not.

You can't believe it, but you left your laptop on the kitchen table last night before you started watching the movie and forgot to pack it. Well, you're fired for sure! You must decide whether to turn back now or push ahead to the airport and hope a colleague has a copy of your presentation and a laptop you can use. What do you do?

The Impact of Stress

Stress doesn't leave our bodies and minds the second we resolve a situation. Instead, we carry it with us throughout our days, months, and sometimes even years. When we're faced with a situation that's unpleasant, worrisome, fear-inducing, or even nightmarish, it feels almost impossible to see the light on the other side. Additionally, stress leaves a mark on us in ways we might not even realize.

Agitation, anxiety, and worry aren't new and unique concepts. We all experience these most days, and even long-term practitioners of meditation and yoga encounter these feelings. The difference derives from our ability to handle such stressors. Over time, our intense feelings create a barrier to our abilities and accomplishments. When we experience difficulties, our fight-or-flight instincts react and we want either to work ourselves into a state of agitated defense or to retreat and repress our negative feelings. Either solution leads to more stress since neither properly acknowledges how to recognize our feelings and calm our emotional state.

When we carry tension or unresolved feelings with us, our bodies and minds are bound to spill these emotions sooner or later. Muscle tension, sleeping problems, gastrointestinal issues, headaches, sadness, or an overall lack of motivation in life are just some of the problematic results of chronic stress (American Psychological Association, 2018). In time, these effects impact our behavior and relationships with others. For example, an individual who relies on smoking cigarettes and drinking alcohol to try to relax is responding to a negative feeling by adding harmful behaviors to their lifestyle.

Understanding that your behaviors may be a response to your emotions is a helpful step in the right direction for making changes to your habits. The suggestions at the end of this chapter will offer some ideas for stress relief, but in getting to the source of a problem, you may need to take more time to reflect on your personal feelings so that these can stop triggering negative behaviors.

Life Experiences

Since we now know the role that stress plays in our daily experiences, we can also relate to the snowball effect these stressors have. In one interesting study in 2013, participants were placed in the mildly stressful situation of having their hands submerged in icy water, and then shown pictures of snakes or spiders (Raio et al., 2013). The stress on the cognitive functions of the participants were heightened with the exposure to an additional stressor, making it difficult to relax from the first one. With this idea in mind, it's easy to see how stress accumulates in our minds, drawing our attention away from other activities, conversations, or projects, adding up in our psyche over time.

Negative experiences related to past trauma carry into our present if we don't have techniques to learn from them. It's important to seek professional treatment if you've experienced a traumatic circumstance and it's holding you back from success. If you believe stress is impacting your ability to work, exercise, or relax, talking with a doctor is an important first step in receiving help and treatment.

Mindful Ideas for Stress Management

Whether facing emotional or physical stress, it's vital to learn about methods you can employ to calm the mind and body so that it doesn't constantly hold you back from living. Techniques for coping with stress and anxiety vary, but taking opportunities for self-care throughout your day will allow you to start forming a habit that's beneficial as you continue to better understand the connection between your brain and body. Choose from the following ideas when you need to release tension or support your practice of self-care.

- Listen to music or podcasts that calm you and make you happy.

- Make your visual world appealing. Hang pictures or paintings you love in your home or office.

- Take a warm shower or bath.

- Use essential oils to calm your system.

- Try a mindful coloring book.

- Start an art project. Paint, sculpt, or build an artistic piece.

- Reorganize one room or area of the home (closet, bathroom, bedside table). Take pride in small accomplishments like this.

- Breathe consciously: try box-breathing, or an exhale-focused breath e.g. inhaling for four counts and exhaling for six counts.

- Take breaks throughout the day to walk around until you feel calm.

- Talk with a friend who inspires you.

- Participate in a community event for charity (do something kind for others).

- Laugh (watch something funny or laugh with a friend).

- Practice yoga or tai chi.

- Keep work separate from your personal space and life (even within the home, have a separate area that's just reserved for work).

- Discuss stressful feelings with a trained professional.

- Consciously relax your jaw throughout the day.

- Create a boundary for your time and stick to this (even when it's hard).

- Allow your body to rest when you're sick. Don't overextend yourself.

- Rethink your day. Before any activity that has the potential to be stressful, think, "What if everything went well?" Walk through the best day you're about to have in your mind.

- Stay hydrated throughout your day.

- Get a plant for your office or home (or both!).

- Sit in a comfortable chair throughout your workday. Proper posture can improve mood.

- Learn to forgive yourself and move on from mistakes. They happen.

- Practice acceptance and kindness daily

- Avoid compulsive behaviors or vices that aren't beneficial.

- Make time for yourself each day (even if it's only 10 minutes).

- Get outside on sunny days.

- Stretch your muscles.

- Eat a fruit you love.

- Take a walk in the park. Observe any sounds around you (birds chirping, the wind blowing through trees, dogs barking, people talking, etc.).

NB: *The above self-care ideas help settle your brain and body for regular mindfulness meditation practices. See Appendix for free audioguides on mindfulness meditations. Use these audioguides alongside the above self-care practices, as you embark on your "Year of Mindfulness".*

Key Takeaways

Naturally, no individual craves an anxious life, but stress can occur with modern life, more responsibility, and previous trauma. Using mindful techniques to place a bookmark in our day, cultivate something nice for ourselves, and re-energize our minds can help mitigate the stress we all experience.

- Stress can stay in the body and mind for days, months, or even years after the experience.

- Recognizing that your feelings can impact your actions lets you take the first step in changing your habits.

- Trauma from the past can impact the present when we don't possess mindful ways to process our feelings.

- Talking with a physician about stress that impacts your capacity to work, exercise, or unwind is a positive step in seeking guidance and treatment.

- Allowing time for meditation breaks during the day can help you establish a self-care routine, leading to a deeper understanding of the connection between mind and body.

In the next section, we'll move to one of the harder ideas associated with mindfulness. When we learn to detach from unnecessary stress and create boundaries, we can find a greater connection to ourselves and those who support and love us.

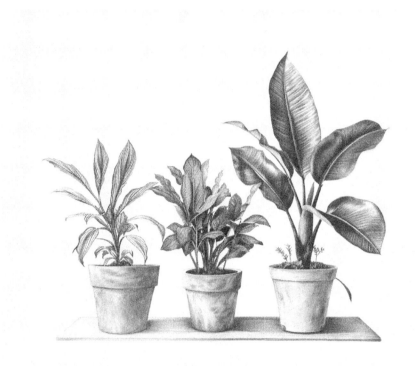

Chapter 6:

How to Let Go with Daily

Meditations

Have you found yourself going about your day when, all of a sudden, there it is—another intrusive thought? *Hurry! Run! Hide!* You think to yourself. But escaping unwelcome thoughts is difficult, especially without the help of a calming practice.

Many of us experience negative or self-critical thoughts. Moreover, we may have people in our lives who add to our stress and meddling thoughts, making even simple tasks difficult. In this chapter, we'll examine how we can alter the way we think about ideas that cause us harm so we can learn to set boundaries with others and become more productive in our daily experiences, alleviating anxious practices and stressful outcomes.

Before diving into this section, though, let's back up for a moment to understand why certain thoughts seem to take hold of us. For the most part, humans are inherently good. We want to help others, show empathy, try hard, and succeed in life. Of course, there are exceptions to this, but I'd guess that the people you know personally in your life are living each day with the intent of doing what they think is right. However, it becomes challenging when a perfectionist mindset, overthinking, or unexpected stress impacts our ability to think clearly.

Imagine a friend texts you to tell you the exciting news that they were just hired for a new job. Depending on where you are in your stage of work or life, you may feel happy for them, but if you happen to be struggling with a job that doesn't feel fulfilling or causes you stress, your response to your friend's news may be shaded with frustration, jealousy, or anger. Most of us don't want to feel this way and many of us will hide any negativity, but it's human to experience a mix of emotions. In some cases, an initial response can fester and lead to feelings of shame, doubt, or insignificance.

So, what can we do personally to take more control of our feelings and the responses we have to ideas and events that arise daily? The concept of "letting go" may not be an easy one to put into practice, but by understanding what it means to have healthy detachments and learning to set boundaries, you'll be on your way to creating a beneficial mindset for yourself.

Healthy Detachment

If you've noticed so far that the concept of mindfulness connects with having a kind of "meta-awareness" of your thoughts and experiences, you're understanding one of the key components of this practice. As we've discussed, the goal within many mindful practices is not to get caught up with emotions or feelings related to the ideas that pop into the mind, and instead to simply observe these thoughts as if we're an outsider to them.

The ability to concentrate on the breath and be a bystander to additional thoughts takes practice, and can be achieved with regular mindful meditation. "While maintaining explicit but minimal focus on the anchor, one uses mindful meta-awareness to sense features of the ongoing experience that are not about the explicit object...but are instead about the off-object features" (Dunne et al., 2019). An example of a "focus on an anchor" might be the focus on your breath or body.

The relationship between having the ability to mindfully watch thoughts float by gives us a foundation for understanding the basics of healthy detachment. Because this practice relies on finding ways to demonstrate kindness to ourselves, it's important to first place this concept at the forefront of the practice. We're not detaching to show malice or coldness to others, rather, we're detaching with a mindful approach for self-care and growth.

"Between stimulus and response there is a space. In that space is our power to choose our response. In our response lies our growth and our freedom."

I love the above quotation, often attributed to Dr Viktor E. Frankl. It is a powerful illustration of the freedom of choice that comes with the practice of mindfulness and healthy detachment. You become empowered with the ability to make conscious choices to your responses, instead of having a triggered reaction. This idea allows a person to search for peace, problem-solving, and move forward.

To discover what you need to detach from, think for a moment about how you might feel stuck throughout your day. Some of us have necessary obligations such as being a caregiver to children or the elderly, so the concept of healthy detachment needs some clarification since our service to others is often required.

Consider which items serve you no purpose and which might cause you more frustration by staying attached to them. When it comes to setting healthy boundaries, consider them for various life categories, such as work, family, home, and relationships.

Work Boundaries

We could have the most amazing jobs and co-workers in the world, but without a separation between work and home life, our minds may continually feel rushed to keep up and complete tasks. Start thinking about the lines you could draw when it comes to your mental energy. It's often difficult to mentally leave work behind once our workday is finished, so establish a transitional way that you can end work so that you're mentally prepared to leave it behind. This could mean incorporating a simple act at the end of your workday to remind your brain that work is finished. For example, turning on a "signal song" that's the same each day or setting a phone alarm to remind yourself that it's time to leave this portion of the day behind.

Creating a work boundary could also mean saying "no" at times. Of course, it is important to contribute to our jobs. At the same time, we also need to communicate to others when we feel overstretched before this becomes a problem where we feel burned out in the workplace. Communication is key here since creating this kind of boundary may require discussions with leaders or bosses, whilst staying clear and honest about why you need to set a boundary is vital. If creating work boundaries is difficult for you, speak with friendly colleagues about the issues you may be having and see if there's a solution you can create together.

The idea in Oliver Berkeman's book *Four Thousand Weeks: Time Management for Mortals* concisely explains the pressure we place on ourselves in trying to accomplish tasks, "Rather than face our limitations, we engage in avoidance strategies in an effort to carry on feeling limitless. We push ourselves harder, chasing fantasies of the perfect work-life balance...Denying reality never works, though" (Burkeman, 2021). When we don't pause to acknowledge our inner thoughts, purpose, or dreams, we deprive ourselves of something greater and operate as simply a cog in a machine.

Family Boundaries

Saying "no" to family members can often be more challenging than creating a boundary with co-workers, so establishing this boundary takes some finessing. If you constantly put up with comments or actions that make you uncomfortable, pause to consider how this is affecting you mentally and emotionally. Without getting upset or argumentative, find a way to communicate how you feel uncomfortable when someone uses hateful or harmful actions or language.

You have every right to protect yourself and those you love from family members who make you feel mentally drained of energy or who don't support your well-being. In your desire to care for yourself, remember that a boundary doesn't need to be permanent, but it can provide you with a break so that you can place your positive energy elsewhere. Stating your feelings to family members is a key part of creating this boundary. It's important to be clear and direct when approaching these discussions but don't point the finger of blame. Calmly explain how you feel and why you have decided this boundary is needed for you.

Home Boundaries

Even living alone can challenge us if we do not have boundaries for our space at home. For example, if your phone, television, or laptop are constant distractions from other activities you could enjoy at home, it may be time to create limits with these barriers that may hold you back from other experiences.

If you find yourself mindlessly scrolling through internet posts first thing in the morning, consider consciously avoid technology for at least the first 30 to 60 minutes of the day. Instead, start your day with awareness of your thoughts and let these guide you to self-discovery. Starting with a short meditation to begin your day can set a tone of calmness for your mind as you embark on whatever the day holds.

If you live with others, creating personal boundaries for yourself at home can prove difficult when noises, conversations, and interruptions are simply a part of your day. If you find that you're struggling to create a boundary for yourself within your own home, communicate your desire to have some time to yourself. Even if you're asking for ten minutes in your day to meditate alone, read a book, take a walk, or exercise by yourself, it's important to express your need to have this time since this can recharge your energy and allow you to become more productive and relaxed.

Relationship Boundaries

One of the most challenging areas of boundary creation comes with making them in our everyday friendships or romantic partnerships. We may feel guilty if we don't have enough hours in the day to spend with everyone. Consider setting aside personal time to complete activities that we want to do or create a boundary with someone who isn't valuing our time or energy.

If you ever feel that you're experiencing mental fatigue as a result of socializing with certain individuals who drain your energy, you might find yourself with a new opportunity to create a boundary.

Setting an emotional boundary for yourself requires taking a closer look at relationships with others. If you're being put down by others or if you regularly have unresolved arguments with a person, it's time to reevaluate this relationship. Is it serving you well? What could you do with your time if you weren't spending it with this person? Is there any hope of the other person respecting a boundary you set with them? Take some time to consider your feelings when you're near this person as well as how you feel when you have time apart.

Boundaries don't need to be permanent, but if you're feeling harmed within a relationship, either mentally or physically, it's time to place an end to this as soon as possible. If you feel you'll need help in creating a boundary with another individual, especially in a harmful relationship with a partner, seek help from a trusted resource such as a family member, valued friend, or support hotline available in your area.

Building relationship boundaries can sometimes be a complex area since it deals with emotions and ideas that may be uncomfortable for some to discuss. Reach out to a therapist or counselor if this is an area that you or someone you know struggle with.

Good books on this topic, such as books by Nicole Lepera and Nedra Tawwab, offer readers guidance on setting boundaries and forming healthy relationships.

Getting Unstuck

In your quest for opportunities to feel productive and detached from activities or people who hold you back from chances to grow, it's necessary to focus on your present situation. Of course, thinking about the future can prove helpful for long-term planning, but encourage your brain to stay mindful of your current circumstances and reality. For example, finding outlets for any anxious thoughts can create a space for them without giving them the power to take over. Start getting your mind unstuck today by reserving five to ten minutes to allow yourself to worry. Really! This may sound silly or even counterproductive, but giving your mind a limited amount of time to think about any stress you're experiencing can feel freeing as you move forward with other more productive thoughts in your day.

In addition, getting "unstuck" might require you to somewhat trick your brain into focusing on a healthier activity such as participation in a sport, crafting, exercising outdoors, or decluttering a closet. Your mind may still wander to a stressful idea, but you can bring it back to making decisions about the task at hand to push the anxious thoughts away.

If there is a problem that needs immediate attention, make the most appropriate decisions to solve what you can, then give yourself a break to focus on an activity that might distract your thoughts from stressful or unnecessary ideas. Instead of thinking about this activity as a way to defer your stress, consider it a method of adding healthy breaks to your day that will offer a release from unwanted thoughts.

Mindful Ideas for Healthy Detachment

When considering methods of boundary creation and ways to make the most of your interests, remember to mindfully step into creating a space for your boundary. If you're breaking away from a person you were once very close to, consider what's changed in your life or theirs that may no longer satisfy you or fill you with joy.

We all have times of self-progress and development, so, at various stages of your life, you might find that you need to pivot so you can care for yourself and separate from any damaging ideas you once gravitated toward. Let this list of mindful ideas for healthy detachment guide you in your search for ways to break from your routine and find moments for yourself.

- Write a list of hobbies you love (or used to love). Try one of these this week.

- Simplify your life. Consider what physical and mental space can you create for yourself.

- Ask yourself: "Is this serving me well?" If not, consider letting this go.

- Find like-minded people that you can talk to.

- Try detaching from social media (even for an hour or two).

- Practice communicating with family members. You shouldn't allow anyone to ignore your needs, but you also need to make your needs known to others.

- Face problems head-on instead of avoiding them or hiding from them.

- Seek professional support to help limit or eliminate your use of alcohol and drugs.

- Observe your thoughts each day. Imagine you're an outsider observing your thinking brain.

- When you experience disappointment, take a moment to reflect on the experience. Give yourself time to acknowledge why you're disappointed, find a way to accept the feeling and then let it go.

- Acknowledge that your feelings are powerful and that you're allowed to feel them.

- Focus on your breath for several minutes to help break the cycle of ruminative thoughts.

- Make space for some "alone time" to reflect on your day.

- Recognize that you can show compassion and understanding without becoming entangled in others' perspectives or conflicts.

- State your needs as specifically as you can.

- Stay consistent with the boundaries you've created.

- Identify any old beliefs that you might need to update.

- Listen to others without judgment.

- Give yourself "time-outs" when you feel anxious or stressed (allow yourself some recovery time).

- Ask yourself, "What is within my control at this moment?"

- Realize that there are many possibilities for outcomes instead of just one. When faced with an important choice, brainstorm all the ideas you can think of.

- Don't wait for happiness to come to you—plan activities that make you happy!

- Ask yourself, "What did I learn from this experience?"

- Reflect on whether specific foods or a lack of exercise might be hindering your ability to detach.

- Set alarms for "mental breaks" throughout your day.

- Practice difficult conversations before having them.

- Wait a moment before answering a difficult question (pause and think first).

- Recognize that past trauma may impact future attachments or detachments. Working with a therapist or counselor can help when unpacking and understanding trauma so that healing can take place.

- Recognize that life doesn't always go exactly the way that we plan, but this is an opportunity for growth and learning. Letting go off old expectations frees us to welcome new opportunities.

NB: The above self-care ideas help settle your brain and body for regular mindfulness meditation practices. See Appendix for free audioguides on mindfulness meditations. Use these audioguides alongside the above self-care practices, as you embark on your "Year of Mindfulness".

Key Takeaways

Understand that there will be ups and downs on your road to mindfulness. Some days, it may feel challenging to create a space where you can observe your thoughts and stay aware of present opportunities. On these days, consider putting on your "emotional brakes" and finding an activity or person to help you reset. The more you take time to make yourself happy, the more natural finding time for this simple act will feel.

- Healthy detachments give a person the opportunity to let go of unsafe or unhealthy relationships.

- Creating a distance from an activity or individual that does not positively contribute to our well-being can be a form of self-care.

- Boundaries with work, family, home, and relationships may be needed to gain a better sense of self-awareness and comfort.

- Remaining in the present moment with mindfulness can help a person adjust to a new boundary.

The next chapter will give you a chance to reflect on your day-to-day routines to see how mindful choices can become more of a natural part of your life. After all, when you learn to live peacefully, you understand how to live mindfully.

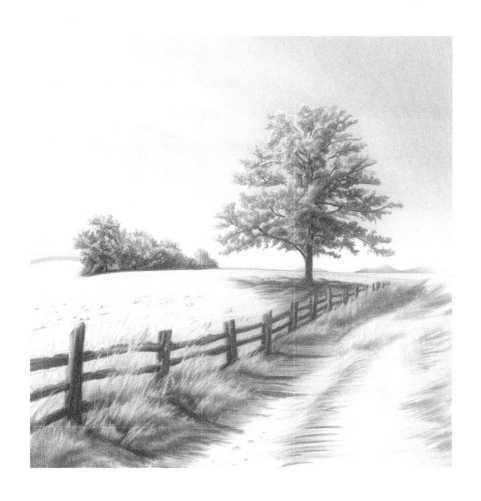

Chapter 7:

Living Peacefully

If you catch yourself feeling envious of the lives of others, keep in mind that the grass isn't always greener on the other side of life's fence. While some days you might not feel like you have it all together, it's important to remember that most adults face ongoing challenges and benefit from both external support and their own mindfulness practices.

Mindfulness has come a long way since its adoption from early religious philosophies. The "no-self" idea of Buddhism traditionally meant that, since a person naturally gravitates toward thinking of themselves first in the world and the items that can become theirs, mindful practices would allow them to settle this craving so that this competitive attitude isn't present (Giles, 2019). Buddhist philosophy encourages leaving behind self-centered ideas like jealousy, envy, and greed so these don't become the focus of a person's life.

While mindfulness in Western culture has many ties to the traditions of Buddhism, the concept of leaving the "self" behind to live a more fulfilling life probably wouldn't connect with an individual who's working to decrease stress. Working to calm the physical body, relieve intrusive thoughts, and eliminate lingering worry tends to mean that we must take an inward approach to deeply understand ourselves and our values.

With this in mind, think of mindfulness as a way to achieve a greater sense of thoroughness in all aspects of our lives. It gives us a chance to walk into any situation with an understanding of ourselves so that we don't have to become someone we're not. The goal, instead, is to recognize our feelings as we mindfully and peacefully live.

Live Peacefully, Not Perfectly

Do you ever catch yourself in a moment of frustration and are not proud about the way you're behaving? For example, if someone cuts you off in traffic, you might find yourself fuming with rage, your heart racing as your hands grip the steering wheel. In many situations, our bodies can tell us a great deal about how we feel without us even having to speak or even think much about it.

There's something to be said for the idea of working toward having more neutral feelings when we meditate or practice activities with mindfulness. Of course, this isn't easy when we have big emotions that can get in the way, but one key idea that can help is to focus, in small ways, on progress and not perfection.

Eliminating the Physical Items

Living peacefully doesn't need to mean that you uproot your life completely and become unrecognizable, but it should mean that you make mindful choices about what you want to keep close to you and what you don't. Start by considering your physical space and any items that may no longer serve you well. Think about what household items and clothes you no longer need and start peacefully living in the mindset that physical items don't equate to happiness. The more we have physically around us, taking up space, the more we tend to feel a crowding inside the mind.

Start mindfully deciding what items around the home or in your closet you could donate to create a clutter-free environment for your body and mind. To paraphrase the concept that Marie Kondo shares in her beautiful book, The Life-Changing Magic of Tidying Up, it can be helpful to consider the question "Does this item bring me joy?" when deciding whether to keep an item.

Eliminating the Decisions

In addition to feeling overwhelmed when our physical space gets crowded, our minds carry stress when we have too many daily decisions to make. This isn't to say that we no longer need to complete necessary chores, but in many circumstances, we add stress to our day with our inability to simplify. When we have too many choices about what to wear, eat, watch, or scroll through, our mind gets overstimulated to the point of feeling lost in the process of decision-making.

Instead of trying to take on all of the activities around you, start making some firm decisions about which activities are necessary and which aren't. The fewer decisions your brain has to make daily, the clearer you'll feel when important decisions arise. Spend your energy in purposeful places and consider what decisions you can eliminate to feel more free.

Your Core Group

When you learned about boundary-setting in Chapter 6, we discussed taking a break from people who aren't supporting your mindful goals. You can explore this idea even deeper now by evaluating who makes you feel valued, desired, and happy so you can create your "core group." Think about who respects your work, time, activities, and other general aspects of your life, and keep these people close. Just as you would want to support others by letting them know how special and valued they are, this core group should be made up of individuals who remind you of how exceptional you are.

A core group doesn't need to be a large group. You can keep this group small since these are prominent friends and family members that you want to spend quality time with. If it helps, create a list of three or four people who you know will support you in both difficult times and successful ones. These people don't have to be friends with one another, but can instead be standalone individuals who will make you feel happy and peaceful.

Understanding Who You Need to Be

Now that you've considered how to establish boundaries as well as create a core group that supports you, realize that, while you don't have to live on an island, sometimes you can! This means you don't need to stress yourself with feelings of guilt or obligation when you have to say "no" to others. Yes, friendship is a two-way street that requires people to extend the support that they'd want to receive, but you should also feel comfortable in making your own decisions about how to reserve time and energy for yourself.

In planning your time with others, save time for yourself. Alone time can be more practical and beneficial than we realize. Most likely, you understand that when you're "on the go" during all hours of the day, you can quickly tire from this unsustainable way of existing.

With this in mind, the practice of mindfulness can help you learn more about yourself and your needs so that you can choose what activities you save energy for and, alternatively, when you need to rest. This idea should make some sense when you think about it—if we try to take on too much, our mental health can suffer, causing anxiety or depressive states. Specifically in studies of the brain, depression can occur as a result of emotions impacting the amygdala due to overactivity in this area of the brain (Barnhofer, 2019). When our stress continues, this area remains hyperactive unless we can make changes to calm it.

Other studies have pointed to the benefits of Mindfulness-Based Cognitive Training (MBCT) in altering brain plasticity for stress reduction in patients (Barnhofer, 2019). These studies' conclusions are meant to give insight into how mindfulness can decrease negative thoughts and improve a patient's mood through mindfulness training since patients can better acknowledge and detach from setback patterns related to stress.

By saving time for mindful practices, we support our brain's health by also allowing it to transition from one activity to the next. This helps with our adaptability in many situations. When we're able to remain flexible, we're also able to build our emotional resiliency, which allows us to cope better in future moments of stress. Yes, we still experience nervousness and worry, but we can remain more fluent as we navigate our world.

A Simple Question

When life feels overly complicated and you need even more managed guidance to gain some control over your path to peacefulness, return to one simple idea. This concept can help you on your toughest days, when working, caring for others, or simply going outside your home feels difficult. Ask yourself, "What do I need most right now?" and wait for your mind to answer this question. I realize this might sound ridiculous, but give it a try the next time you're spinning out of control. Sit in a quiet location, close your eyes, take a deep breath, and ponder this question to see what happens.

I've found that when I've tried asking myself this and waiting for an answer, something definitive eventually pops up. Your brain will know what you need when you need it. Sometimes, my brain wants me to sit longer to meditate while I calm myself down. Other times, my mind gives me a single calming affirmation like "I can do this," which powers me through the rest of my day. Occasionally, my brain tells me to indulge in something that's kind for my body, like a bath. Whatever comes to me as I sit tells me that's what I need, and allowing myself to have that is a gift to myself.

Try it the next time you need a release. Simply ask yourself, "What do I need most right now?"

Mindful Ideas for Peace and Resilience

Remember that taking time to remind yourself of what you love in life can help you stay rooted in the present moment. As you consider adopting the items below to your life, you may want to find a journal or notebook to keep track of your path to peace and resilience. Begin by writing down a few things that you're grateful for at the moment so you can start by creating a habit of appreciation.

- Make a list of five things you've accomplished or tried for the first time so far this year.

- Adopt a kinder, more compassionate view of others, whether you know them or not. Practice being non-judgmental and try to be curious about others instead.

- Show yourself kindness with a non-judgmental attitude of yourself.

- Simplify your life by decluttering areas of your home.

- Spend time in places that you love in your home.

- Get outdoors. Go on new adventures.

- Try using blackout curtains in your bedroom. This can help you enjoy a better night's rest so you wake feeling refreshed.

- Invest in a cozy blanket or comfortable sheets (or both!).

- Try writing down the simple pleasures from your day (eating delicious healthful food, trying something new, complimenting someone, etc.).

- Acknowledge yourself for activities, skills, or hobbies you *can* do, and not to get caught up in what you can't do.

- Recognize that you won't be in the same stressful moment forever (everything is temporary).

- Track any triggers that might upset you and reflect on what you can do about this.

- Keep a calendar or to-do list of your "top five" necessary tasks each week.

- Add variety to your life (take a new route to work, try a new food, listen to new music).

- Join a group or club that you're passionate about.

- Make a list of role models in your life. Journal about the qualities you admire in them.

- Laugh and keep a sense of humor throughout your day.

- Stay flexible and adaptable when events don't go your way.

- Take time to prepare and practice speeches and presentations.

- Be aware of the number of times you check personal emails or text messages throughout the day.

- When you're stressed, try using essential oils or lavender scents to calm you.

- Take a bubble bath.

- Paint or color a picture.

- Take a "mini-vacation" for a weekend by yourself.

- Use a soothing lotion before bedtime.

- Write a journal entry about something that angers you, then tear up the paper and throw it away. Imagine that this is unnecessary anger that you're ridding your life of.

- Reserve at least one day a month to stay at home and recharge your energy.

NB: The above self-care ideas help settle your brain and body for regular mindfulness meditation practices. See Appendix for free audioguides on mindfulness meditations. Use these audioguides alongside the above self-care practices, as you embark on your "Year of Mindfulness".

Key Takeaways

Continue identifying the positive aspects of your life and writing these down as a quick list that you can glance at in difficult moments. When you're able to appreciate the ideas and items you're grateful for, it becomes easier to feel a sense of accomplishment for the life you've built for yourself.

- In Buddhist philosophy, mindfulness focuses on eliminating self-serving concepts like jealousy, envy, and greed and instead encourages a separation between such feelings and the human mind.

- Eliminating physical items and decisions that no longer serve you can help you focus on a stronger sense of purpose. In addition, choosing a core group that supports you can help establish a connected relationship with encouraging friends and family.

- Mindful practices alleviate stress and overstimulation of the brain so that the mind can detach and start learning healthier habits during difficult setbacks.

We've come to a pivotal point where we can begin to narrow our focus on some of the aspects of life where mindfulness may come in handy most. Since a workday can become one of the most anxiety-inducing aspects of life if we allow it to be, we'll now discuss how to manage and take control of this portion of our day with grace and readiness.

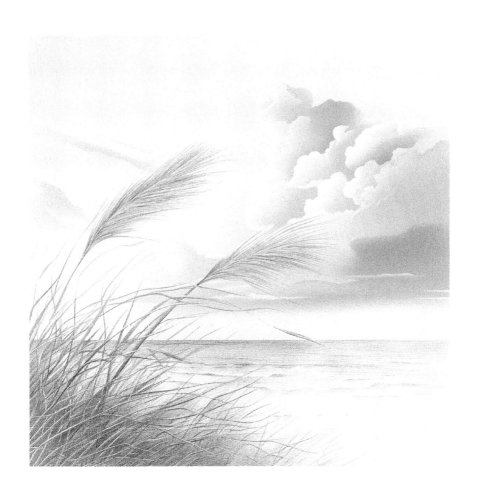

Chapter 8:

Conscious Breathing for the

Workday

If you could make one wish about your job or workplace right now, what would it be? Would you want to have a higher paying salary? Would you wish for a kinder, more understanding boss? Would you want coworkers who value and appreciate your efforts each day?

Most of us dream about improving at least one aspect of our work life, but changing anything about a job can be challenging and feel out of our control. So many people crave a work-life balance that allows them to split time equally between the job and fun so that they don't carry the weight of work into their personal lives. But is this even possible in a Western world that thrives on industry and productivity?

Sadly, "40% of workers reported their job was very or extremely stressful" and "25% view their jobs as the number one stressor in their lives (Batson, 2021). Evaluating happiness during a workday sounds subjective—and to some degree, it is—but with this statistic in mind, most of us cannot deny that working a stressful job is no one's idea of a perfect day.

In this section, we'll explore how to decrease feelings of stress in the workplace and beyond. With conscious breathing techniques, we can better recognize when we feel anxious about work and learn to take breaks to recharge at these moments. We'll also talk about ways to better balance life and work so that the latter doesn't become the larger portion of our day. While most of us consider work a necessary part of our lives, there are ways to improve our thoughts about work so that its challenges become more productive learning opportunities.

What Is Work, Really?

In understanding the concepts that this chapter will present, I realize that the word "work" could feel limiting. After all, what is work? We all have "work" we need to accomplish, right? This simple word contains many meanings and for some, can have a negative connotation. By rethinking and redefining "work", we can explore this in new ways. While many of the ideas presented here could relate to a nine-to-five job, they could also connect with any tasks that feel necessary each day.

Since there are all types of jobs as well as people who work to complete these jobs, it's first necessary to describe the varieties of work because each has its significance. Managers of major companies work to ensure that employees are completing tasks and are satisfied in their roles. Entry-level employees at a company work to gain experience and learn how to lead. Trainers at a gym work to build relationships with clients so they'll feel motivated to work out. Unpaid caregivers work to assist loved ones in times of need and dependency. Stay-at-home parents work to make difficult decisions for their families each day. Regardless of the type of "work" you're a part of, you make a difference in the lives of others and need support and nourishment to continue doing so.

Because it's obvious that the idea of "work" doesn't make everyone immediately excited, identifying any problem points or areas for improvement needs to be a first step toward feeling satisfaction with work. While doing this doesn't need to be a monumental task, it is an important beginning for understanding how to change or adapt to work situations. Just as with other areas of our lives, we need a sustainable experience so we don't burn out too quickly when it comes to work.

Take some time to examine your current situation and any parts of it that you think could be better. What would it take to improve? What conversations would you need to have? How do you think these conversations would go? If there are any lists you need to make in this process, now is the time to pull out some paper or a notebook to jot down ideas. There are no wrong answers in the brainstorming process, so feel free to list anything that comes to your mind while evaluating your experience of work.

Evaluating Work Stress

Imagine having a job where you're able to wake up in the morning after a great night's sleep, experience eight productive hours of uninterrupted workflow, and then end your day doing activities that you enjoy without even a hint of a reminder of your job. Yeah, right. If you're rolling your eyes at this point, so am I—this feels like an impossibility for any line of work.

An important question to start asking yourself is, "What makes your job particularly stressful?" You might have a laundry list of examples to answer this, but let's start focusing on the top one or two for now. If you had a chance to journal about what might improve your job, feel free to use an idea or two from this list. In reality, you could probably categorize work stress into one of the following areas: the physical, the emotional, and the organizational. Most likely, any source of stress that you list could fall into one of these categories, so take a moment to decide what categories your top examples fall under.

To more deeply understand what implications each category could have, we'll now examine some examples of stress in these categories.

Physical Work Stress

The physical stress from a job can add up exponentially. This category tends to be one of the more stressful when you focus on the sustainability of a job. For example, if you lift heavy objects, endure loud sounds, or work in poor lighting throughout your day, the stress from this is likely to physically affect your body over time.

Emotional Work Stress

Question: What's sometimes more difficult to deal with than the physical stress of a job?

Answer: The emotional toll it takes.

When considering workplace aggravators, psychological stressors like harassment, poor working relationships, burdensome job demands, or mental anguish all impact an individual's emotional well-being. Some people might brush this off as "just part of the job", but it's important to take a closer look at what results factors like these cause over time as a person may discover that their career may not be worth long-term harm.

Organizational Work Stress

The organizational stress in a job tends to be a bit more subtle but can creep in as time passes. If the management structure of a workplace causes harm over time to employee output, everyone suffers. While this kind of stress can impact a person emotionally as well, its cause is rooted in the inadequacies of a company as a whole. For example, if employees aren't given the proper tools to complete a job, stress can develop. Sure, employers may spin this lack of resources as a way to have employees show their ingenuity and creativity, but there are numerous other ways to allow employees to demonstrate these skills while also meeting their basic needs. An organizational culture that encourages open communication and trust, and support staff wellbeing can benefit both the company and the employees.

Job Insight

As you well know, the impact of having a job doesn't just weigh on a person at one particular moment. We accumulate stress as it snowballs from one task to another, so it's important to have tools to combat this stress before it gets out of control.

If you've ever experienced a job where there's a high turnover rate, poor employee morale, or excessive absenteeism, you have probably taken some time to contemplate whether this job is worth continuing. In mulling over your decision, understand that you're not alone and that someone, somewhere is feeling similarly.

Even in your most stressful moments with your job, remember that, in most cases, you still have a choice in the outcomes that occur. Even in instances where a person feels stuck in a job that causes stress, they can still make decisions about how they will proceed. In some cases, this could mean leaving the job completely, but it doesn't have to. Having an important conversation with others about work-life balance, job stressors, or the physical demands of your day can lead to a change in confidence and production at a job.

Giving yourself more insight into how you feel about the work you do each day can offer you the knowledge you need to make some of the challenging decisions about what to do next. Consider your answer to the following questions and your rationale behind each response:

- Do you feel significant in your workplace?

- Do you feel you play a direct role in the success of your work?

- Do you have cordial relationships with co-workers?

- Are you involved in decision-making at your workplace?

- Do you want to be involved in decision-making at your workplace?

- How do you feel about working in your current job five years from now?

While there are ways to make significant changes in our lives every day, sometimes small changes are all we need to motivate us momentarily.

This can be enough to get us through the day and refresh ourselves for upcoming tasks.

To become more mindful throughout your day, find time to practice deep breathing exercises for a few minutes at a time. Just as you would in your home, find a quiet, comfortable place to sit and relax for a few moments. If you can, dim the lighting or close your eyes and concentrate on breathing in and out to relieve tension.

In this next section, you'll learn several specific ways to release stress through breathing techniques that can quickly calm you. Try these at a desk, on a lunch break, or when you simply have a quiet moment during your day. These exercises won't take long, so any amount of time you can make for them during your day can help you relax.

Conscious Breathing Exercises

The idea of focusing on the breath can sometimes feel like an annoying exercise in futility. We sit there, inhaling and exhaling, while trying to focus our attention on our breathing. How many times have you felt distracted and defeated by this exercise? After all, the mind was meant to think, and it wants to have something to do at all times of the day while we're conscious.

To alleviate any stress you may have experienced in the past when focusing on the breath, there are several ways to experiment with conscious breathing during meditation or other activities.

One idea for conscious breathing includes the process of silently counting from one to ten with each breath you take. This can give the mind something to focus on and turns your brain to an activity that's simple, yet centered on one task. Once you've reached the number ten in your mind, you can then count backward from ten to one while syncing the number with each breath. Do this for as long as necessary so that you can place your concentration somewhere while still eliminating serious and unnecessary thoughts from the mind.

According to *Harvard Business Review*, adding focal exercises throughout a workday can improve productivity and attention when it's time to plan, organize, or create, leading to better focus for employees. In addition, the two defining skills in mindfulness are "focus" and "awareness" since these areas will present a departure from interruptions of the mind (Hougaard & Carter, 2016).

When practiced both at home and in the office, mindful exercises like conscious breathing bring a release to our day so the rest can feel purposeful and effective.

Anchor Breathing

One type of conscious breathing to try both in and out of the workplace is the technique of anchor breathing. This kind of breathing allows a person to fully concentrate their thoughts on their breath, or "anchor" thoughts so that the mind is absorbed in a scenario that leads to a mellow outcome (Celestine, 2020). You could imagine you're relaxing on a soft towel at the beach on a warm summer day. You can feel the ground beneath you and you feel connected to the Earth. Or you can simply notice the sensation of the breath. You may wish to lay down, close your eyes, and place your hands on your stomach; breathe in and out slowly and feel your stomach rising up and down as you breathe. This is your anchor point. Concentrate your focus on this movement and breathe in and out for a few moments to feel relaxation.

Box Breathing

A method known as box breathing allows you to gain relaxation by breathing in, holding a breath, and exhaling for a certain number of seconds. This breathing technique can quickly and easily bring a sense of peace and comfort to the mind. The exercise can be done in many places such as while sitting in an office chair or on a park bench.

Typically, box breathing invites participants to breathe in for four counts, hold for four counts, and breathe out for four counts, and hold for another four counts before repeating this sequence. This calming breath gives you a chance to concentrate on the counts within your breath instead of getting distracted by your surroundings as you work to settle your mind.

The 4-3-7 Breathing & Cyclic Sighing

One of the most calming breathing techniques is breathing which focuses on longer exhalations.

One of these is the 4-3-7 breathing technique. This means that you take a breath in for four seconds, hold it for three seconds, and exhale for seven seconds. There are variations for the duration of inhale, hold, and exhale, e.g. 4-7-8. The key is the extra-long exhales. These long exhales let go of tension and activate the parasympathetic ("rest and relax") part of the autonomic nervous system. I also recommend a pause for a few seconds after the long exhale, before repeating the next cycle. As you perform this exercise, imagine your stomach as a balloon that you're trying to deflate as much as possible as you exhale the air in your lungs. Repeat this breathing technique for a few minutes at work or at home to settle your mind or before transitioning to a new activity.

Another is cyclic sighing, also called the physiological sigh. With cyclic sighing, first take a full inhale, then take another sniff of breath; it may help to feel the sides of your ribs expand further with this extra sniff of breath. Next, take a slow and long, extended exhale. Cyclic sighing can improve mood and reduce stress (Balban et al, 2023).

I have found these two breathing methods which focuses on slow extended exhales, to be effective and easy to share in my clinical practice.

Mindful Ideas for Productivity

While any job can have its ups and downs, it's necessary to rely on tools that will help you feel more relaxed and productive each day. Evidence suggests that practicing mindfulness can assist individuals in their workplace and lead to results such as positive social behaviors, authenticity, creativity, and leadership (Rupprecht et al., 2019). When we invest in and rely on mindful practices to guide us throughout our day, we open our minds to more opportunities.

The following ideas can offer ways to treat yourself to mindful practices before, during, or after work, so don't be afraid to try something new.

- Stay open-minded with others at work. Avoid judging their work or situation.

- Explore new ideas at work with colleagues by asking questions, planning a walking meeting or seeking mentorship from someone you admire in your profession.

- Create a quiet, calm space for yourself no matter where you work (home or office, outdoors or indoors).

- Set a time to end your work each day. Make a point to "close your workday" and continue again the next day.

- Remember to take a regular break from your screen, every 30-45minutes and move your body. Take a walk, do some stretching, make a hot drink – this will help reset your mind ready to return to the task at hand.

- Create a priority list at the start of each week and plan out what needs to get done when – anything non-urgent can be put on a separate list to work through if you have the time after the urgent tasks..

- Add a gratitude practice to your work day. Consider three things you are grateful for about your job, your company, your industry or your colleagues.

- Encourage yourself and others to participate in self-care activities both in and out of work. This helps foster a culture that values self-care.

- Pack healthy lunches and snacks for work that won't make you feel sluggish throughout the day.

- Set an intention at the start of each workday. What do you hope to accomplish?

- Take a quick meditation break at work (find a quiet space and use headphones to block noise if needed).

- Realize that some workdays will be better than others. Challenges and failures will occur.

- Use a comfortable chair for work (if you sit for your job).

- Limit multitasking whenever possible.

- Set phone alarms to take "meditation breaks" (even just for a few minutes at a time).

- Seek out professional help when needed. Speak to your manager if things are getting too much and talk with a counselor about job-related stress issues.

- Actively listen to others at work. Request that others do the same for you.

- Seek opportunities for growth (continue learning even if you've done the same job for a long time).

- Show respect for others. You'll find that others will respect you as well.

- Don't wait to tell colleagues about a job well done. Thank people for their work, even if it's small jobs, and you'll soon notice people will do the same for you.

- If you work from home, create a 'transition' task to signify to your mind and body that the work day has ended. This could be going for a walk, making a tea, putting on some favorite music – anything that encourages that switch-off.

- Timebox conversations about work outside of work when socialising, whether with work colleagues or other friends and family. Set a time limit for everyone or each other to talk about work so it doesn't dominate all the other great things you have to share and talk about.

- Create incentives and rewards for yourself for completed tasks.

- Recognize and take comfort in the routine of your day (drinking coffee, attending a morning meeting, eating lunch regularly).

- Don't be afraid to change jobs (or careers) if something isn't working out. Seek advice on how to transition to something else.

NB: *The above self-care ideas help settle your brain and body for regular mindfulness meditation practices. See Appendix for free audioguides on mindfulness meditations. Use these audioguides alongside the above self-care practices, as you embark on your "Year of Mindfulness".*

Key Takeaways

Remember that work in any form may not always be easy, but with added strategies for brain health, you can carry these tools both into and out of your workday to feel a sense of control and relaxation.

- Evaluate what qualifies as "work" during your day. What jobs have you taken on in your life?

- Recognize what stressors you experience at work each day. Make a list of these. Decide what is physical, emotional, or organizational stress.

- Work to understand what makes you feel challenged, positive, negative, lonely, powerful, or any other emotion during your workday. With insight into your feelings at work, you can add mindful practices at stressful times.

- With mindful breathing exercises like anchor, box, 4-3-7 and cyclic sighing, you can employ quick, calming techniques that are practical for relieving tension during the workday.

As you know, stress can cause a ripple effect in other areas of life. Difficult emotions not only arise in the workplace but also in the home, leaving a damaging impact on our bodies. When stress occurs, one of the most vulnerable areas becomes our digestive system. In the next chapter, we'll look at the important role of proper digestion in our lives.

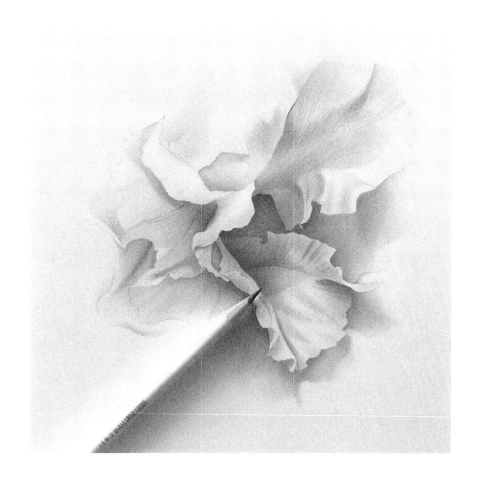

Make a Difference with Your Review

Share the Gift of Mindfulness

"The greatest gift you can give someone is the gift of peace of mind." - Unknown

Dear Reader,

Congratulations—you're more than halfway through this book! Which parts of this book do you find particularly helpful so far? I hope you don't mind this pause in the book's flow with this little message.

Have you ever noticed how sharing something meaningful with others brings its own sense of calm and satisfaction? Just as mindfulness helps us find peace within ourselves, helping others discover this path can create ripples of positive change.

Would you help someone who might be feeling overwhelmed, anxious, or stuck in patterns of overthinking – someone who, like you, is seeking a way to find more peace in their daily life?

My mission in writing "Mindfulness for Brain Health" was to make mindfulness accessible and practical for everyone who wants to experience more peace and joy in their daily lives. Through actionable strategies and practical techniques, this book offers a path to better brain health and emotional well-being, especially for those feeling overwhelmed by life's demands.

Many people, when feeling overwhelmed or stressed, turn to books for guidance. They often rely on reviews from readers like you to help them choose their next step. Your honest review could be the gentle nudge that helps someone take their first step toward mindfulness.

It takes just a minute of your time, but your words could help:

...one more person discover lasting peace and joy
...one more overthinker find freedom from anxious thoughts
...one more individual transform their relationship with their mind
...and create ripples of positive change in our community.

To share your experience and help others, simply follow the link or scan the QR code to your local Amazon marketplace to leave a review:

USA Amazon.com/review/create-review?&asin=1738558118	UK Amazon.co.uk/review/create-review?&asin=1738558118

CANADA Amazon.ca/review/create-review?&asin=1738558118	AUSTRALIA Amazon.com.au/review/create-review?&asin=1738558118

Or search your **Local Amazon Marketplace** and enter
ASIN=1738558118
or search "Mindfulness for Brain Health by Dr Sui Wong".

Thank you for being part of this journey of bringing more mindfulness and understanding into the world. Your support means more than you know.   Mindfully yours, Dr. Sui Wong

With shared gratitude and presence, let's return to our mindfulness journey together...

Chapter 9:

Digestion and You—A Mindful

Approach to Weight Management

Here you are again, faced with the decision of what to eat. You could choose something healthy, but you're starving and feel like vegetables and fruits won't satisfy you. You could stop off at your favorite pizza place on your way home from work, but is that the best choice today? Will it make you feel good to scarf every slice within 10 minutes while watching TV?

Why does it always feel like we only have a few moments to eat a meal from start to finish? Are we so busy during the day that we can't take time out to sit down and eat? If you're yelling, "Yes! I am, in fact, that busy!" I'm right there with you.

While taking a mindful approach to eating sounds like an impossibility, it's something we can all make time for, we just need to know how. The age-old question of what to eat so often stresses individuals and families, leading them to choose fast, unhealthy meals that cause weight issues, illness, and gastrointestinal problems. What we often ignore, though, is how significantly digestion relates to our emotions.

It's time to take control of the foods you eat by making more mindful choices. You're already on your way to learning how to do this by acknowledging the other areas of your life that may need more mindfulness. In this chapter, you'll discover non-strenuous methods of heightening your food awareness so you're able to eat consciously and care for your body and mind.

Mindful Eating

Let's begin this conversation by synthesizing the basic idea of mindfulness presented in this book so far. If you've noticed one thing about the practice, it might be this—it's not a process that should be rushed. Truly take a moment to think about this. Is the fastest way always the best way? We tend to think so in this eat-or-be-eaten, reach-the-top-first society, but when it comes down to it, slow and steady pays off—especially with mindful practices.

Because mindfulness requires a person to focus on their awareness and present situation, the practice of mindfully eating closely relates to this intention. Making thoughtful choices of what to eat as well as sitting down to slowly absorb the process of eating creates a more mindful experience overall. "Mindful eating encourages one to make choices that will be satisfying and nourishing to the body. However, it discourages 'judging' one's eating behaviors as there are different types of eating experiences" (Harvard School of Public Health, 2020).

With this in mind, think of how many times in your life you may have thought, "I hate myself for eating that." The idea of mindfully eating isn't a free pass to eat whatever you want, but it will challenge you to stop and ask yourself more questions before consuming your food. To start putting this into practice the next time you're hungry, pause for a moment and ask yourself:

- Am I hungry or bored?

- Could I find an activity that would take my mind off eating or do I truly need food at this time?

- What food will make me feel healthy and energized three hours from now?

By creating this awareness of your feelings about the situation, you're removing the quick, mindless process of stuffing food into our bodies quickly just because we can or because we feel we have no other option.

"Mindful eating stems from the broader philosophy of mindfulness, a widespread, centuries-old practice used in many religions. Mindfulness is an intentional focus on one's thoughts, emotions, and physical sensations in the present moment" (Harvard School of Public Health, 2020). By keeping the present moment at the forefront, you're automatically arming yourself with an incredible ability when it's time to make and eat a meal or snack. After creating an awareness of how hungry you're feeling, decide what foods are right for you at that moment. While this could occasionally mean that a cheeseburger or ice cream is right for you in moderation, choosing a healthier option may satisfy you just as much and keep you powering through your day for longer.

The point is to slowly and consciously begin to think about foods differently. Consider every aspect of eating a meal from start to finish. Think about where the foods are coming from, how much you enjoy or don't enjoy the foods you've chosen, and what your body will feel like after eating. When we take time to consider this, we slow the process that we've grown accustomed to and have a chance to enjoy the foods we're eating.

Now, I know what you're thinking. You might wonder how "slowing down" anything is possible when, on most days, you're working to keep yourself and possibly others on track. As with any long-term goal, start small with this one, too. You don't need to uproot your entire existence and change everything about the way you've always eaten, but you can start the process by channeling an awareness about your eating habits. Taking a closer look at the simple act of when you eat and how you eat can tell you a lot about your habits.

One of the main steps in increasing awareness of mindful eating habits is by paying closer attention to the foods we eat. When shopping for food or selecting meals at a restaurant, it's important to sit with the options for a moment and think. Consider what will satisfy you most and improve your eating experience. Again, some days, this may mean indulging in foods that may not be quite as healthy as other ones, but try doing this mindfully and use your senses to experience the food. Slow your eating process by taking time to first look at and smell the food. Wait several minutes before tasting it. Appreciate the way the food was prepared for you or the way you prepared the meal you're about to enjoy. Using physical and emotional senses to enjoy food allows you to have a much more mindful experience of eating so you can remain in the moment while eating rather than reacting to your state of hunger (Harvard School of Public Health, 2020).

Weight Management

When learning to mindfully eat, consider educating yourself on healthy food options that can allow your body to feel its best. I'm a firm believer in the idea that mindful eating can lead to healthier food choices, so while the ideas in this section are not necessarily with the goal of weight loss in mind, they will provide some guidance that could result in weight loss due to eating healthier foods slowly and consciously.

The ideas here are meant to encourage weight management through the creation of healthy habits and routines. "Intervention studies have shown that mindfulness approaches can be an effective tool in the treatment of unfavorable behaviors such as emotional eating and binge eating that can lead to weight gain and obesity" (Harvard School of Public Health, 2020). By starting to instill healthy habits for eating today, you pave the way for a process of mindful growth for yourself. Deciding what to eat while keeping in mind what you *should* eat isn't easy, but consciously creating opportunities for your brain to make purposeful decisions about food helps reinforce a better approach toward eating.

When making conscious food choices, remember to:

- Schedule routines for eating.

- Avoid excessive snacking, but eat when you're hungry.

- Store healthy foods around the house and at work.

Having a routine when it comes to eating can ensure that your mind doesn't panic when thinking about when your next meal will come.

When leaving the house, consider packing a healthy snack so you're not caught without something to eat.

For some, skipping meals can lead to excessive hunger and overeating, which can hinder efforts of more conscious eating. However, it's also important to make decisions about eating because you're hungry and not force yourself to have a snack just because you feel you have to. Consider pre-planning some easy and healthful go-to snack or meal options, for when you're hungry.

Lastly, keeping healthy foods stocked in your pantry and refrigerator can eliminate some of the tough decision-making when you find yourself hungry. Try packing a lunch for yourself before you leave the house for work, and include foods that will satisfy your appetite so you'll stay full longer. Packing fresh fruits, vegetables, a healthy protein like beans, peanut butter, or hummus, and a grain like whole grain crackers or pasta can help keep your energy up as you continue the day (Harvard T.H. Chan School of Public Health, 2019).

Preparing meals for the week ahead of time, such as on the weekends, can also add an element of mindfulness to your eating. If you buy the ingredients and create healthy packed lunches for the week ahead, you're likely to spend time more time considering what foods you should put into your body rather than quickly eating fast food because you're short on time during the day. If you have a family, consider making meal preparation an activity you can all participate in on the weekend to help each other pause and think about what you would like to eat throughout the week.

Mindful Ideas for Healthy Eating

Practicing mindfulness while eating stems from an awareness of the experience of eating in considering what's best for our bodies. Start listening when you feel full, sick, or hungry so that you can make appropriate choices when it comes to eating and living better. "Combining behavioral strategies such as mindfulness training with nutrition knowledge can lead to healthful food choices that reduce the risk of chronic diseases, promote more enjoyable meal experiences, and support a healthy body image" (Harvard School of Public Health, 2020). By understanding your current habits with food, you can make more informed decisions about how you'd like to make and eat meals each day.

The following mindful ideas for healthy eating can help when thinking about foods and forming new habits.

- Slow down while eating or drinking.

- Create a "food schedule" and stick to eating at these times.

- Bite and chew slowly and thoroughly.

- Consider the source of your foods. Where are the products coming from? Are they natural? Does the process of making them help or harm the planet?

- Research the restaurants you go to and the foods you buy.

- Always consider how your body will feel after consuming the foods you're choosing.

- Avoid eating on the go or in the car whenever possible. Make eating an event and sit at a table to enjoy your meal.

- Eat vegetables before the rest of the meal.

- Consume at least one green vegetable each day.

- Let yourself stop and think for a moment when you're hungry to consider what foods would satisfy you most.

- Breathe in and out after each bite.

- Prepare more meals at home.

- Talk to others about any tips they use to prepare healthy meals.

- If possible, avoid getting too hungry or too full.

- Prepare and carry healthy snacks when traveling (dried fruits, nuts, veggies).

- Drink lots of water each day to stay hydrated.

- Consider if you're eating because of boredom, e.g. ask yourself, "Am I hungry?"

- Avoid watch television or a movie while eating.

- Put your phone away during mealtimes.

- Eat with family and friends. Savor the experience.

- If you overindulge, it's not the end of the world. Try not to feel guilty and instead simply try again.

- Use your senses to experience the look, smell, sound, feel, and taste of each food you try.

- Cook and try new foods that you've never eaten before (our palates need variety).

- Appreciate the foods you're able to eat (practice gratitude).

- Make a food journal entry about the favorite foods you ate within a day, week, or month. Write about how they made you feel.

- Put your utensils down between bites. Take your time with the meal.

- Evaluate which foods make you feel your best and which make you feel sick or tired.

- Realize that your eating experience is unique. Find foods that will healthily satisfy you.

NB: *The above self-care ideas help settle your brain and body for regular mindfulness meditation practices. See Appendix for free audioguides on mindfulness meditations. Use these audioguides alongside the above self-care practices, as you embark on your "Year of Mindfulness".*

Key Takeaways

Remembering to focus on one task at a time can be difficult for many, but this is one vital step in mindful eating. When you're able to slow down, think, and make clearer decisions about food, you're able to tune in to what you truly need and can eliminate damaging distractions.

- Make mindful eating decisions by slowing down the process of making and eating meals. Absorb the overall experience of eating.

- When deciding when and what to eat, ask yourself if you're hungry or bored, if another activity could take your mind off eating, and if the foods you're choosing will replenish nutrients and energize your body.

- Consider packing healthy snacks and meals when you leave the house. Schedule times to eat throughout the day so you don't allow yourself to get overly hungry.

Since decisions about eating will need to fit your lifestyle, remember to make a schedule that's practical for you. On hectic days or when you're stressed, try taking a few deep breaths and thinking about what will make you feel best in the moment. Start listening to this inner voice to guide you in other areas of mindfulness, as well.

The next chapter will help you focus on an aspect of life that many struggle with when stressed. The process of sleeping presents challenges, but learning to train the brain with mindful practices to prepare for a healthy sleep routine sets us on the right path toward recovery.

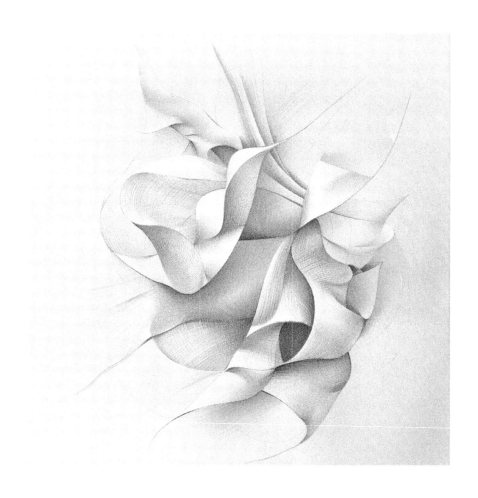

Chapter 10:

Sleeping with Peace and Purpose

When you were younger, were you able to fall asleep fairly easily? Did you nap on long car rides in the backseat or fall asleep in a parent's arms at restaurants? The ability to easily nap changes dramatically as we age. While we may realize that sleep is important, we also tend to experience new forms of sleep once we're teenagers. The sleep habits we build during these years don't do us many favors as we get older and often can pave the way for poor sleep routines into our twenties and beyond.

Establishing bedtime routines as a child helps individuals extend this practice throughout life, allowing for the development of proper patterns in falling asleep, staying asleep, and remaining alert throughout the day from early childhood (Pacheco & Callender, 2021). As teenagers and adults, we forget this, though, and might view the act of staying up later as exciting. After all, we feel like we can be more productive because we're completing more activities if we limit our sleep, right? At some point, however, sleep deprivation catches up with us, and we need to improve sleep patterns to stay healthy.

Healthy sleep habits can impact working memory, cognitive abilities, mood, and attention overall. It's not surprising to hear that the ability to regulate stress levels is linked to positive sleep habits, but we may not understand how to change these if we've been practicing poor sleep habits for so long. Introducing mindfulness can alter the way we view this process and help us enjoy better nights of sleep.

Why Sleep?

We know we need sleep, but why is it so important for our bodies and brains to get regular, scheduled sleep throughout our lifetime? Well, our bodies and minds are much smarter than we know. For example, have you ever relied on muscle memory for a workout or dance routine? You'll surprise yourself with just how much your body and brain are connected as well as how practice over time enhances our abilities in almost everything. I figured this was the case when I began my journey to find better sleep, but I didn't expect to find that quieting my mind and body while I slept would improve my ability to learn and remember, as well.

Allowing our bodies to sleep consistently offers other benefits for our minds as well. Matthew Walker who has done tremendous work in advocating sleep to the public, and written an eloquent book "Why We Sleep" (2018), shared this in 2006:

> This 'offline' effect can restore previously lost memories or produce additional learning, both without the need for further practice. In other words, the enhancement phase of memory consolidation is an active process, not merely one of simple maintenance; the brain continues to learn even though it has stopped practicing.

Earlier, when discussing the brain's cognitive functions, we talked about how, while unconscious, the brain doesn't have as many opportunities to cling to new information. This idea still stands, but the sleeping brain reveals much that we can learn regarding the way we perform and function each day. A lack of regular sleep increases our risk of illness and disorders like heart disease and dementia and, in addition, mood overall is impacted, says National Institute of Health sleep expert Dr. Marisha Brown (Wein, 2021).

While restorative naps can help manage sleep for short periods, damage from a consistent lack of sleep leads to problems over time. Because our sleep works with our system's hormones, metabolism, and immune system, it's suggested that the average adult needs at least seven hours of sleep within twenty-four hours (Semeco, 2017). When we don't receive this much sleep, our cognitive functions are thrown off, and this can be difficult to recover from. Consider the last time you didn't sleep well and how this made you feel the next day. Your mental well-being throughout the day might have felt more negative than usual, and you may have found yourself making more mistakes, too.

As you know, your memory helps you function at work, in social situations, and independently when you're on your own. When memory is affected by limited sleep, the active process of recalling information can't make as many important connections within the brain. For example, when we don't sleep for long periods consistently in our twenties, we might become more forgetful with simple tasks throughout the day. We may forget to take out the trash or call a friend back on the phone—things that seem like minor oversights, but forgetting many of these small tasks adds up quickly. This can make us feel somewhat out of control during the day, but we may not make the connection that a lack of sleep and our forgetfulness are related.

As we age, our internal clock changes, and we tend to get fewer hours of sleep due to our bodies' circadian rhythm (Walker 2018). This can feel stressful, but there are ways of getting a good night's sleep that don't have to feel overwhelming. With mindful and calming practices, it's possible to retrain the body so that a positive sleep routine can take priority.

The Practice of Creating Calm

While you probably realize the importance of sleep, you may still struggle to find opportunities for regular sleep since this tends to be one of those areas of life that fluctuates. You get busy during your day and need to spend extra time at night catching up on chores or work. You stay up later on weekends since this might be your only opportunity to do so. You may even make a point to get into bed earlier some nights, only to lie in bed for hours frustrated that you can't fall asleep.

It's time to end the sleepless nights by creating a routine habit of calm before, during, and after sleep occurs. It's important to remember to speak with a physician if you feel you've tried all methods of falling asleep quickly and soundly, as there may be other issues that need addressing, but for most people, incorporating a few essential sleep practices will improve rest. For more on this, access the bonus content in the appendix.

Incorporate Physical and Mental Activities

Each day, it's important to stimulate the mind and body. Exercising isn't just for our bodies as it also creates a chance for our minds to participate in a rigorous activity that will help us sleep at night. Your physical activity of choice doesn't need to be strenuous as long as it challenges you in new and interesting ways. For example, simple stretching before bedtime can lead to better sleep. Walking, jogging, lifting weights, or riding a bike can provide opportunities to burn energy that our body is storing so that we become more tired at night. In addition, try not to exercise late at night as this impacts the sleep cycle and the body's circadian rhythm. It's best to exercise in the morning to stimulate the mind and body for the rest of the day. You don't have to push yourself to participate in something you don't like, but try creating a weekly workout plan with the activities you'll complete so that your physical energy is expelled.

In addition to the physical practice of releasing energy, our mind often needs to be challenged mentally to feel tired at night. Burning mental energy by playing a game that requires strategy, socializing with others, reading new information, or producing an artistic piece allows the mind to feel like it's had a brain workout. Now, suppose you're already busy and challenged by tasks throughout the day—you might already feel exhausted by the end of each day. In these cases, you don't need to add more. Otherwise, consider adding brain stimulating activities during the day that gets your mind working so it can rest when needed.

Find Comfort

Just like children, adults need cozy, comfortable atmospheres and objects to promote sleep. If you've spent the night in a place that's made you uncomfortable, you know how difficult it can be to sleep. The goal of finding comfort for sleep is to make the physical environment and aesthetic atmosphere as comfortable as possible so you can settle your mind and sleep. Make your bed a place of relaxation, in fact, allow your entire bedroom to become this, as well. Some find it helpful to leave televisions and electronic devices outside of the bedroom so that it becomes a sanctuary for sleep and intimacy only. You might consider this as you search for ways to mentally and physically alter your sleeping habits for the better.

When our bedroom feels soft, safe, and pleasant, our mind will start to make the connection that this is an area for relaxation. After a short time, you may even find yourself yawning or feeling sleepier as you enter your bedroom since this location has a specific purpose.

Put Away Electronics

As mentioned, electronic devices typically don't do us any favors when we're training our minds for sleep. Set a timer on your phone at least one hour before bedtime to remind yourself to start getting into "sleep mode" for the night. While this idea isn't a revolutionary one, it will remind you each night to make sleep a priority so your brain sees it as one. Even on weekends, place your phone or laptop aside as you settle down during the hour before bedtime and notice how much this can change your ability to fall asleep. Reading or writing before bed can create a sense of calm as well, so these may be great alternatives to using a phone.

Limit Eating and Drinking

I know, I know. This one sounds like no fun, right? But by limiting the amount of caffeine, alcohol, and food we have before bedtime, we can create a night of more restful sleep. If you've relied on alcohol to help you fall asleep in the past, you'll know how this might have worked briefly, but you most likely didn't stay asleep for very long or receive a restful night's sleep.

Using caffeine in the afternoon may give you energy to power through the rest of a workday, but it can affect your ability to fall asleep by the time bedtime rolls around. Limiting or eliminating caffeine in the afternoon, sets us up for a better night of sleep. Matthew Walker often shares in his interviews, that the quarter life of caffeine is 12 hours, i.e. approximately 12 hours after consuming a cup of coffee, a quarter the amount of caffeine is still in your body (Walker 2018).

Finally, eating or overeating near bedtime can also affect you getting the complete rest you need. Symptoms of indigestion and heartburn can keep a person awake and feeling ill while trying to fall asleep. It's best to finish eating for the night several hours before bedtime to ensure that digestive issues won't keep you awake.

Mindful Ideas for Improved Sleep

When considering what mindful steps may be right for you in assisting with sleep, remember to try strategies that help you relax and not feel overstimulated before bedtime. While the ideas below provide a list of options, listen to your body and brain when they're telling you to slow down and relax. A night of rest can feel restorative and therapeutic, so work to create a calming routine that places your needs first when it comes to sleep.

- Sleep regularly. Get to bed around the same time each night and wake up around the same time each morning, even on days when you don't have to leave the house early. This will help you establish a routine.

- Remove electronic devices from the bedroom at night.

- Finish eating about three hours before bedtime.

- Avoid alcohol and try not to eat at least three hours before you want to go to sleep. Both of these can cause inconsistent and disrupted sleep.

- Avoid caffeine, including chocolate, late in the day. Caffeine and sugar are both stimulants or the mind so, as above, can lead to disrupted or difficulties sleeping.

- Meditate before bedtime. See the appendix for a free bonus guided practice.

- Take a bath or shower before bed.

- Listen to soft, slow music at night.

- Gently stretch for a few minutes before bed.

- Read a chapter of a book before trying to fall asleep.

- Journal about your day before bedtime to calm your system and reflect on events.

- Set your phone to sleep mode to avoid texts, calls, and emails while asleep.

- Use soft and low lighting at least one hour before bedtime.

- Keep any pets off your bed as you try to sleep.

- Avoid naps after 2 p.m.

- Don't force sleep. If your mind is anxious before bed, walk around for a few minutes or journal your thoughts to calm yourself.

- Avoid watching the clock while in bed.

- Include exercise in your day, but don't exercise too close to bedtime as this can disrupt the process of relaxing before bedtime.

- Wear cozy, soft clothes before bed to set a mood of comfort.

- Light a scented candle (but don't fall asleep with this candle still lit) or use aromatherapy to promote sleep.

- Find the right sleeping position for you. Evaluate sleep when you're on your back, side, or stomach. What allows you to relax the most?

- Get enough sunshine or bright light exposure in the mornings. This can help when it's time to transition to low lights before bed.

- Practice relaxation techniques such as deep breathing or progressive muscle relaxation before bed to help ease your mind and body into a state of calmness.

- Visualize your favorite vacation spots or calming locations while trying to fall asleep.

- Research and practice some yoga postures that promotes better sleep.

- While in bed, try tightening all your muscles for a moment, then relaxing them to settle your body.

- Wear comfortable pajamas to bed.

- Try using a weighted blanket to feel protected and safe while sleeping.

- Change your mattress or bedding if you feel these aren't comfortable enough for proper sleep.

NB: *The above self-care ideas help settle your brain and body for regular mindfulness meditation practices. See Appendix for free audioguides on mindfulness meditations. Use these audioguides alongside the above self-care practices, as you embark on your "Year of Mindfulness".*

Key Takeaways

As we age, the habits that we've established early in life continue to shape our adulthood unless we take time to create new patterns. The sleep practices we start now can alter previous habits to ensure we get on track to sleeping better, which positively impacts memory and health.

- Creating a bedtime routine each day gives our body and mind a pattern to follow so that we can enjoy proper sleep.

- Inconsistent sleep patterns can lead to higher risks of illness and disease.

- A lack of sleep can affect the brain's memory functions including recalling or retaining information.

- By mindfully engaging in creative activities, designing a comfortable environment for sleep, limiting electronics, and reducing the amount of food and drink consumed before bedtime, the brain can properly prepare for sleep.

Since you now have additional ideas for mindful practices throughout your day and night, it's time to touch on a point that draws many to a life of mindfulness. Treatments for pain are vast and can feel frustrating when the options aren't working as quickly as we'd like them to. In the following chapter, we'll make some connections to the mindful ideas you're now aware of and put them into practice when working to manage physical pain.

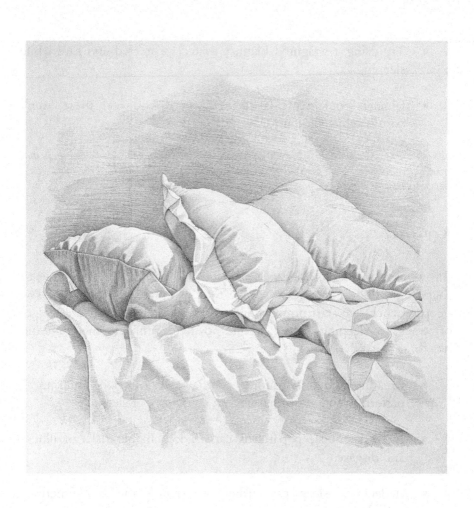

Chapter 11:

Pain Management and Relaxation

for the Body

The challenges we face daily can create mental hurdles, but we can improve our ability to cope with them by practicing mindfulness techniques. But what happens when our pain is a physical one that's more difficult to shake? What if we've turned to doctors, surgeons, and medications, but the pain is chronic and relentless?

Many live with daily physical pain that seems untreatable and causes substantial emotional stress. If you're currently experiencing chronic physical pain, you understand the toll this can have on your life. If you don't experience this regularly, take a moment to remember the last time you strained a muscle, and then imagine this pain remaining with you for years, even decades.

Often, chronic pain leads to damaging psychological results as well, such as depression, anxiety, reduced mobility, or isolation (Reid et al., 2015). While the information in this chapter is not meant to replace medical advice from a physician, it will provide you with potential hope that relief from and management of pain is possible through mindful healing practices.

The Truth About Pain

"No pain, no gain." "Pain is beauty." In our culture, we hear pain frequently associated with something positive that will lead us to a fulfilling outcome. But many of us are raised with an understanding that to be important, strong, or valued, we need to stay silent in our struggles. In reality, a very small percentage of individuals will find success living this way.

At any age, pain that lingers over time presents challenges, but chronic pain tends to impact specific populations more significantly than others—the elderly, women, those who've experienced trauma, and individuals of lower economic status (Reid et al., 2015). While experiences with pain differ in each individual, anyone seeking pain management or relief knows what it feels like to encounter discouraging setbacks almost daily. It becomes difficult to experience life the way others do, and conflicting feelings of jealousy or resentment of those not experiencing pain may start to take hold.

As you've learned in previous chapters, the brain and body have a powerful connection. When negative self-talk takes hold due to pain, it's difficult to draw ourselves away from these feelings. "Nociception is the physiological processing that facilitates noxious information, which at some point in the process becomes the conscious experience of pain" (Grant & Zeidan, 2019). Over time, this stored negativity is almost impossible to release without the help of outside assistance to relax tension. This is where mindfulness can offer relief and support.

With the incorporation of mindful practices, the brain can find connections to positive experiences, even while experiencing chronic pain. Researchers are discovering that pain can be reduced when individuals have positive expectations of an experience (Atlas et al., 2022). For example, if you're expecting pain from falling on the ground, you'll probably believe that you're hurting more afterward than if you didn't approach the fall with this idea in mind. The brain changes and adapts to its circumstances, and the concept that it will alter as a result of positivity or negativity has led researchers to make some interesting conclusions about the brain's receptiveness to mindful practices.

Mindfulness and Neurological Disorders

While the brain often tells us to push forward and continue working at all costs, it's important to know that this philosophy is counterproductive for most individuals, especially those experiencing a neurological disorder. The ability to calm the mind through relaxation exercises that create awareness helps to strengthen the brain's attention in the present moment, which can allow pain or symptoms of neurological disorders to dissipate.

Studies on the impact of mindfulness on individuals with neurological disorders indicated that mindfulness practices can improve a person's quality of life since the brain can be strengthened like a muscle (Grant & Zeidan, 2019). When a person focuses the mind on practices such as yoga, meditation, or tai chi, they nurture the brain and allow it to concentrate on a skill, distracting it from pain and negativity. Participants who suffer from headaches, epilepsy, neurodegenerative disorders, functional neurological disorders, strokes, or movement disorders, and even caregivers of those with neurological disorders, have found relief through mindful and meditative techniques (Kraemer et al., 2022). The result of these studies grounds itself in the idea that symptoms associated with neurological dysfunctions can be reduced to improve a person's general well-being. More research is needed to understand and gain access to spreading awareness of the benefits of mindful practices, but these results provide much-needed hope for anyone suffering from neurological disorders.

I am also excited to share my recent research using mindfulness as a treatment intervention for a neurological disorder called visual snow syndrome, a condition due to brain network dysregulation. Our study showed that eight weeks of intensive mindfulness training can lead to changes in brain networks as shown on functional magnetic resonance imaging (fMRI) and improvement of the condition (Wong et al 2024). This study is also promising as a proof of principle, that mindfulness interventions can lead to improvements of neurological conditions through changing of brain networks.

Hope for Pain Management

With chronic pain, an individual's life is often put on hold. Simple tasks or activities that they once enjoyed may no longer feel possible, causing mental stress and anguish. Because we know that the brain is a powerful organ, however, we can now start to understand, through acceptance and commitment, how we can regain the control we once had.

One of the best ways to find relief from chronic pain is to educate yourself about the type of pain you're experiencing. Seek advice and explanations from medical professionals and read about the experiences of others with similar symptoms. Most likely, there's a community of individuals who deal with the same or similar pain, so find support from these people and realize that you're not alone in your struggle. Speak with physicians about pain relief options and stay patient as you test possibilities for yourself.

If a medical professional recommends physical therapy, remember to stay consistent with the exercises you're encouraged to do. One of the fastest ways to relapse during recovery or with chronic pain is to ignore the practices recommended by professionals. While giving yourself time to heal, it's vital to work muscles near pain sites so that these won't atrophy while you wait for any pain to subside. Since the recovery process can be slow, motivate yourself with small goals during this time and celebrate your victories, regardless of how trivial they seem.

Alongside your work with healthcare professionals, you may also find it helpful to explore self-management techniques through breath and bodywork. Jill Miller is a yoga teacher and fascia expert I greatly admire and have had the privilege of learning from over the years. She is the author of two books I regularly recommend: *Body by Breath* (Miller, 2023) and *The Roll Model* (Miller, 2014), that share practices that can ease pain.

Body Scans for Pain Management

In Chapter 4, I mentioned my admiration for Jon Kabat-Zinn and how he first brought mindfulness into the medical context. He developed the Mindfulness-based Stress Reduction program that has helped many people overcome chronic pain (Kabat-Zinn, 2013). One of the components of this program is a bodyscan practice.

Participating in body scanning practices requires a sense of open-mindedness for individuals who suffer from pain. As you might be aware from yoga and meditation practices, concentrating on deep breathing and examining the brain's thoughts from an objective point of view can be challenging. Body scanning asks an individual suffering from pain to engage in a similar practice but to concentrate on parts of the body to relieve pressure and discomfort.

Body scan is a mindfulness practice where the individual zooms in on parts of their body, bringing an openness, curiosity and relaxation whilst exploring their pain. The technique is usually guided by another individual who asks a person to close their eyes and concentrate on breathing in and out deeply and mindfully. After several minutes of this, the facilitator will guide a person to focus their attention on an area of the body. When the mind wanders, the participant is gently encouraged to bring their attention back again to the body. After several minutes of exploration, the individual can open their eyes again and notice how they feel. An added benefit to participating in this type of body scanning is that, according to neuroscientific research, focusing awareness on the body and breathing repeatedly helps create new pathways in the brain, which builds our inner strength and resilience (Sevinc et al 2018) .

Pain Reprocessing Therapy

In addition to body scans, about 98 percent of individuals who experimented with Pain Reprocessing Therapy experienced relief from chronic back pain (Ashar et al., 2021). With this method, sufferers became free or nearly free of pain after just four weeks of treatment. Pain Reprocessing Therapy teaches participants about what their brain and body experience when they feel pain so that they can alter their perception of this pain and reduce their fear surrounding it. Think of this method as a type of "mind over matter" thought process. As a patient learns more about the pain they experience, this knowledge takes the power away from their fear of the pain and puts them back in control of their life.

Mindful Ideas to Assist with Pain Management

While pain management can feel like a lifelong process, it's necessary to remember that each time we participate in an activity that feels therapeutic and relaxing for our body, we're also relaxing the mind in the process. Use the following ideas as a way to find relief from any pain you experience while taking care of your mental health. Once you find an activity you enjoy, repeating this can help the mind return to a place of comfort again and again.

- Practice deep breathing exercises to relax the body.

- Try daily stretching or yoga.

- Complete a body scan meditation. Concentrate on the places where pain is felt. Imagine the pain moving out and away from the body. Access my free bonus body scanning via the appendix.

- Try acupressure or acupuncture with a licensed professional.

- Rub essential oils on your neck, temples, chest, or feet for relaxation (lavender, rosemary, peppermint, and eucalyptus are great for pain relief).

- Take a warm bath. Soak for about 15 minutes in water that's between 90 and 100 degrees Fahrenheit (32-37 degrees Celcius).

- If you experience chronic headaches or migraines, try applying cold gel packs to the face for relief.

- Strengthen the muscles that surround the areas that are in pain.

- Self-massage any painful areas (sore feet, legs, wrists, jaw muscles, or neck muscles).

- Practice qigong or tai chi for pain relief. These both focus on slow body movements to improve focus and release pain.

- Talk to a therapist about your pain. Cognitive behavior therapy (CBT) can help provide relief from chronic pain since a therapist can help shift one's perspective on pain.

- Try soft tissue therapy. Speak with a physician about this method of managing various types of pain.

- Engage in progressive muscle relaxation, a technique involving tensing and then relaxing different muscle groups sequentially, proven to alleviate stress and promote relaxation.

- Use soothing hypoallergenic lotions to soothe muscles.

- Avoid sensory overload by taking frequent breaks from electronic devices.

- Take time for yourself. Look around and note your surroundings, ambient sounds, and the way you feel.

- Distract yourself with a new hobby or activity.

- Learn more about your specific pain. Many hospitals offer classes or workshops about various chronic pains.

- Talk with your family members so that they're aware of your pain. Communicate your needs and tell them how you feel when you're facing a painful episode.

- Avoid fatigue due to chronic pain. Try taking a nap or resting before feeling worn out.

- Drink water to stay hydrated.

- Try a cold compress that you can store in the freezer. This idea is especially helpful for headache relief.

- Drink a soothing herbal tea like chamomile.

- Get fresh air each day (go outside!).

- Create friendships with other chronic pain sufferers or attend a support group for pain management.

- Remain proactive with your pain. Don't wait until the pain is unbearable to seek help.

- Stay positive and hopeful that your pain will diminish or end.

NB: The above self-care ideas help settle your brain and body for regular mindfulness meditation practices. See Appendix for free audioguides on mindfulness meditations. Use these audioguides alongside the above self-care practices, as you embark on your "Year of Mindfulness".

Key Takeaways

When a person can finally face any fear of pain or gain an understanding of what types of pain they're experiencing, the pain loses its power over that individual. With this in mind, know that support is out there for any type of pain a person could experience, both physical and emotional, so seek help and treatment sooner rather than later.

- Physical pain and emotional pain can often go hand-in-hand. It's distressing to our mental health when managing physical trauma, whether it's short or long term.

- Muscle tension, anxiety, and depression can result from physical pain since chronic pain lingers in the body and mind.

- Mindfulness provides relief for chronic pain sufferers and leads to an improved lifestyle through the support and relaxation of the body.

- Physicians can provide information about which pain relief techniques and mindful practices may be best for various forms of pain.

- Guided methods like body scanning or Pain Reprocessing Therapy help pain sufferers acknowledge their pain and work to reduce or eliminate it.

- Mindful practices can provide relief to individuals with neurological disorders

Since the experience of pain varies for each individual, it's important to examine and explore what might be right for you and your own needs. As we continue to keep self-care at the forefront of our minds, remember that any progress requires consistency and endurance—two traits that you're learning to master.

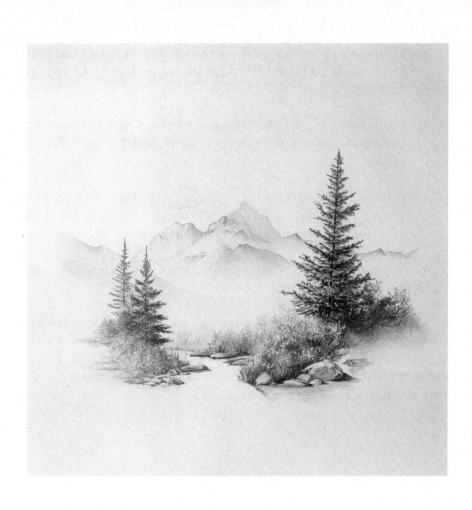

Chapter 12:

Athletic Mindfulness

Even if you don't consider yourself athletic, imagine that you're an advanced swimmer standing at the edge of a lap lane, about to dive in to race against other swimmers. You smell the chlorine as you look forward toward the end of the lane, where you'll need to swim fast. *I've got this!* After all, you know what you're doing. You've trained for years to feel confident at this moment. Nothing's stopping you from this experience—until you take a look around.

All eyes are on you.

You see your friends and family members behind you, and even though they're cheering you on, you can't help but feel nervous. *What if I have a bad race? Will I let everyone down? Why are they all here to watch me? Who am I? Surely, there are tons of other swimmers out there that they'd like to watch more than me?* And just like that, you're absorbed in negative thoughts, doubting your own worth and expertise.

We all experience the dreaded imposter syndrome, even if we're not Olympic athletes. We hear that voice in our head that wants to hold us back from applying for that top job, asking someone out on a date, or swimming with confidence across that pool. While this isn't a unique feeling, you may notice throughout your day that others seem to have it all together without experiencing signs of this setback. But you have to ask yourself, do they *really* never feel fear, or do they simply have tools to cope with feelings of uncertainty?

Well, imagine if you had these tools, too. While athletes work to overcome obstacles by training to be their best selves in both body and mind, this technique can apply to anyone working toward achievement. Athletes around the world work hard physically, but what many athletes don't discuss enough is the role that their attitude plays in their daily routine. Whether you're an avid athlete or want to have the motivation of one, in this chapter, you'll learn how to rewire your brain and open yourself up to gain confidence and participate in opportunities you might once have shied away from.

The Mind of an Athlete

Do you remember the first time you tried cooking, dancing, folding laundry, or typing on a keyboard? It's likely that you weren't excellent at these tasks immediately and that it took some time to get the hang of them. Even if you don't recall the process it takes to gain knowledge and muscle memory, your brain automatically references your previous experience with the skill to perform activities each time you try them. "Due to neuroplasticity, every time a skill is performed our brain refines that motor pathway...If a bad movement pattern is performed repeatedly, the technique will require more practice and time to fix/refine" (Dobbs, 2018). You'll notice this happening if you train to play a sport or work out in a gym but don't feel as if you're making any progress over time. Often, this is where coaches and trainers come into play since they teach us about the proper techniques and insider tips for making improvements.

Since the process of learning and practicing a skill is familiar to all of us, not just athletes, let's talk about how motivation and mindfulness factor into training the brain athletically. Yes, being an athlete takes hard work and dedication to a craft, but staying focused and eager to continue performing is one of the most necessary skills to develop. And how does an athlete build their focus and eagerness? Well, even the toughest athletes often embrace mental awareness as a way to release thoughts and tension before, during, and after a performance.

The Misperception of Athletic Mindfulness

While the public perception of athletic endurance might still be that athletes are strong in every way and don't become stressed since they've trained vigorously for so long, this is simply not true. Understand that an athlete was also once a small child who experienced vulnerabilities just like the rest of us, navigating a world that often feels cumbersome and scary. Like others, athletes experience a wandering mind, stress, and defeat, especially if they've been practicing their craft for a significant amount of time. They question their own strength and stamina, and they have great days as well as rough ones.

So, what's the difference between a person who has out-of-control feelings and nonstop stress and an athlete who thrives in their comfortable zone of wellness? For starters, athletes are often taught how to bring their minds back to their present moment and stay engaged, rather than focusing on mistakes that have happened or could happen. For trained athletes, the ability to process what's happening at the moment and release any stress or tension is a practiced skill that can often take years to master.

Non-athletes can learn this skill as well so they can refocus during times of nervousness or even crisis. Similar to athletic setbacks, we all experience moments when we wish we could push past our fear to exude confidence, or at least appear at ease. What makes the difference in our ability to remain poised and level-headed is found in the key preparation we do between the pivotal seconds of performance.

Consider this—if you just sat on the couch all day watching television and eating pizza and ice cream, would you become a world-class soccer player? Most likely, you're telling yourself, "No." But let me pose this question instead—if you were late to work after a doctor's appointment where you were diagnosed with high blood pressure and you dropped and cracked your phone while spilling soda all over your desk, causing your keyboard to spark and your laptop to be ruined, would you still feel ready to pull off an amazing presentation in front of your entire company? While this case may be extreme, it's an example of how we so often place ourselves in situations without slowing down and mentally preparing our minds to deal with whatever comes our way.

For athletes, the key to creating the feeling of motivation comes with the help of four mindset procedures that help them reset between games or even in the middle of one. These steps include deactivation, reaffirmation, refocusing, and reactivation (Ivey et al., 2015).

- **Deactivation:** This mindful pause asks an athlete to take a few seconds to let go of any negativity or worry associated with their current performance. An athlete can imagine their defeatist attitude floating away or getting squashed like a bug, just as long as the feeling leaves their system.

- **Reaffirmation:** After deactivation, athletes then remind themselves of words or phrases that make them feel positive and strong. Saying something simple such as "I can do this" or "I am strong" can help an individual remember the positive mindset they want and need to have.

- **Refocusing:** This concept places the athlete back in control through the process of visualizing what the positive outcome will look like and trusting that this will become the reality.

- **Reactivation:** Finally, this step asks the athlete's mind to return to the game or performance so that the next part of their execution of skills can take place.

Mindfulness techniques offer athletes valuable tools for both physical and mental recovery. One such technique is the body scan, where athletes systematically direct their attention to different parts of their body, noticing any tension and releasing it. This practice fosters relaxation and aids in the recovery of fatigued muscles.

Additionally, incorporating mindfulness into exercise routines enhances the benefits of physical activity. Mindful exercise involves paying close attention to bodily sensations, movements, and breathing patterns during workouts, promoting a deeper connection between mind and body.

Breathwork techniques are also a great addition to athletic routines. They can significantly enhance athletes' focus and recovery. By practicing mindful breathing exercises, athletes can regulate their nervous system, reduce stress, and enhance oxygen intake, thereby optimizing performance and supporting faster recovery times.

By integrating these techniques into their training regimen, athletes can not only accelerate physical recovery but also cultivate mental resilience, enabling them to perform at their best while maintaining overall well-being.

Visualization for Athletes

If we compare meditation to playing a game, it's almost like the game of pretend that we often play as children. Let this idea be comforting as you explore all the ways you can imagine scenarios to provide comfort and reduce stress. As a child, inventing stories when you played pretend with friends had no limits. You could be a knight fighting an evil dragon or an employee at an ice cream shop that has every flavor imaginable. Allow your adult mind to operate the same way when visualizing success for yourself. The sky is the limit—nothing is holding you back!

Since we've come to realize the power that imagination and hypothetical outcomes can have for an individual, particularly athletes, we can now discuss some of the best visualization techniques to increase awareness and improve performance. The concept of visualizing a positive performance can have as strong of an impact on the brain as meditation, body scanning, and mindful breathing, so it's another area that athletes shouldn't overlook.

For the perfectionist in all of us, visualization offers an outlet for real results. If you can imagine a scenario playing out in your mind, you'll be able to better handle it in real life. Visualizing outcomes can also help us improve memory since we may be running through the same positive scenarios over and over again. To visualize an outcome that you'd like to see, first find a quiet location and sit up straight in a comfortable chair. Slowly and consciously breathe in and out to calm your mind, and imagine the details of the scenario you'd like to picture. Allow this to not only motivate you as your mind walks through this situation but also let this be your practice for the big event. Imagine how the scene will play out on "game day" and try to picture every minute of the performance. Focus on staying alert and relieving any stress now in preparation for the real day. Many athletes find that the process of visualization before the event can decrease the amount of pressure they face during the live experience since they'll already be familiar with the way it plays out (Straw, 2023).

Mindful Ideas for Body Performance

In any performance-type scenario, there will be pressure to complete an activity with perfection, but try to let this idea go as you gather your tools to do the best you can. A benefit to practicing mindfulness is that you won't necessarily need to place a tremendous amount of pressure on yourself anymore since you'll feel prepared for anything that comes your way. The following ideas can assist an athlete in their work toward progress.

- Mindfully breathe (practice this before and during an activity).

- Complete body scans to help you relax. Close your eyes and focus on each part of the body individually, relaxing from toes to head.

- Visualize your success as an athlete before any performance— find a quiet space, close your eyes, imagine the details of a game or event, and visualize your success and the emotions associated with the event.

- Journal daily! Write about your hopes, fears, and successes as an athlete.

- Remember to stretch (before and after each performance).

- Participate in a supplemental physical activity that will assist and enhance your main sport or activity. Examples of this could include yoga, ballet, walking, a kickboxing class, or lifting weights.

- Make a list of the top three goals (in order) of what you'd like to accomplish athletically this year.

- Think of one positive affirmation for yourself and say it aloud each day.

- Learn to leave any failures behind (consider them learning opportunities). State verbal forgiveness aloud after any mistakes.

- Participate in activities that require and build mental focus, such as reading, writing, or painting.

- Record and watch your performance. This can be difficult for some but is worth a try to make improvements. Use this as a learning tool for your training.

- Separate yourself (create boundaries!) from athletes or individuals who speak negatively about their performance or the performance of others.

- Set a personal intention at the beginning of each practice. What do you want to learn or gain?

- Rest consistently and regularly.

- Create a training calendar and post it somewhere prominent so you can hold yourself accountable for practicing.

- Take a warm shower or bath to relieve tension and stress from exercises.

- Try a cold shower to invigorate your body and to practice controlling your breathing throughout the process.

- Listen to music that feels inspiring or motivating to you.

- Watch a favorite clip of an athlete you admire.

- Create a workout habit. Even if you show up to train for just a small amount of time, focus on "showing up."

- If something isn't working, update or change your practice plan. Stay open and adaptable.

- Eat enough healthy foods to properly nourish you for your performance.

- Drink approximately 11-15 cups (91-125 ounces) of water each day to hydrate your body and mind (Eby, 2023).

- Yawn or laugh before a performance to calm any nerves.

- Create a gratitude journal about your body (Example: "I'm grateful for my legs because they allow me to walk and run," "I'm grateful for my eyes because they let me see the goal").

- Find a coach or friend who can positively boost your confidence during practices or on performance days.

- For team sports, participate in workshops or meetings that can build camaraderie with teammates.

- Make a list of the intrinsic rewards you receive from playing this sport or participating in the activity.

- Show compassion and kindness while performing (to others and yourself).

- Practice Progressive Muscle Relaxation (PMR). Slowly focus on tightening one muscle for 8-10 seconds, then relax it. This helps relieve tension all over the body even if you aren't experiencing muscle pain (Toussaint et al., 2021).

- Feel your feelings! You don't need to stop your mind from experiencing certain emotions, even during games and performances. With time and meditative practice, you can simply feel your emotions and move on.

NB: The above self-care ideas help settle your brain and body for regular mindfulness meditation practices. See Appendix for free audioguides on mindfulness meditations. Use these audioguides alongside the above self-care practices, as you embark on your "Year of Mindfulness".

Key Takeaways

While athleticism requires strength and ability, much of this comes from within. Even if you feel that your athletic days are over, possessing an athletic spirit doesn't have to end. Continuing to stay mentally aware and mindfully prepared should be just as much a part of a training routine as exercise is.

- The brain tries to recall prior information to perform tasks, so gaining muscle memory is just as important as strength training for the body.

- Athletes experience setbacks and have vulnerabilities, but they often work to overcome challenges by training the mind for positivity before, during, and after a performance.

- Four practices can assist in bringing athletes back to a state of awareness and focus: deactivation, reaffirmation, refocusing, and reactivation.

- Visualization techniques can be a powerful addition for athletes, on top of mindful breathing meditation, and body scanning.

We've finally reached a point where we can start using some of the mindful techniques we've learned to take our practice to another level. Examining ways to both parent and age gracefully can be challenging, but with the ideas you've gathered, you can apply the practices to best suit your life and needs.

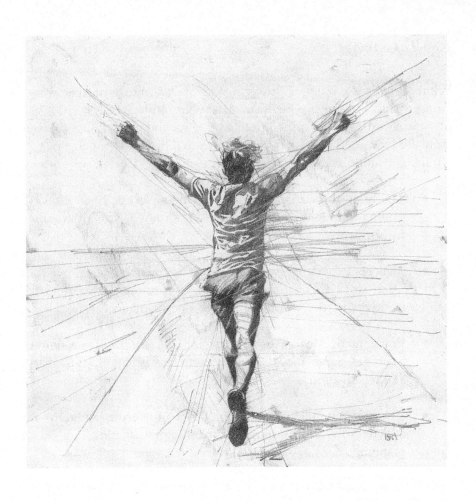

Chapter 13:

Parenting Mindfully

It's another bright, sunny day and you're about to pick your child up from elementary school. As you pull your car into the parking lot, you take a deep breath and realize this will be the last time you're alone for the rest of your day. You savor this moment of quietude. *That's okay, though*, you think as you wave to your child, who walks over to the car and gets in. As you greet them, they let you know that they've had a busy day, but that it was great and they're glad they can relax now. On the drive home, you both enjoy the time together and the space to breathe while calmly discussing your days. You're both present in the moment and can mindfully share your feelings.

If you're a parent, does this sound like a typical day for you? While parenting can be a wonderful endeavor, I'm guessing this hypothetical scenario seems unrealistic in comparison to what you normally experience. Regardless of your child's age, you most likely navigate curve balls with them daily, and by the end of your day, it probably feels like you've experienced more than you thought you would when you woke up that morning.

Parenting in a relaxed and mindful way doesn't have to seem so far-fetched, as the mindful techniques we've already discussed can help us react more appropriately to anything life throws our way. The act of parenting is something to be admired. It is also a tough job. Maybe you've experienced this yourself and lost your cool during an interaction with your child. While this is nothing to be ashamed of, know that there are mindful approaches you can use to tackle everything life throws your way.

Mindful Stages

Mindful parenting consists of pausing to consider the choices and reactions you're having to situations with your child, which is something few of us tend to do when our days are busy. Staying present is hard when we're juggling meals, car rides, homework, diapers, or tough conversations with kids. This requires staying conscious of what's happening now so we don't miss opportunities or get upset when something isn't going our way.

You've now gained insight into some tools that will help you stay mindful, so in this section, you'll learn how to carry these methods into your life while parenting. Being a parent is an important job, so you'll not only have a chance to focus on what's right for you but also what's necessary and helpful for your child. It's never too early to practice mindfulness or to teach a child how to stay mindful throughout their day. As you read, consider ways that you'll be able to achieve mindfulness as a parent through the help of these powerful methods.

Mindfulness for Infants

Arguably, one of the most challenging aspects of parenting is communication. When we care for infants, the fact that they can't speak to us to describe their emotions or pain can be frustrating for us and for them. It's up to us to decipher what an infant needs based on their body language, cries, and facial expressions. By practicing mindfulness, we can develop the skills to understand our connections with others, even infants.

An important activity for childhood development is the "back-and-forth interactions children have with caring adults. [In addition,] building our capacity to be fully aware in the moment allows us to become more attuned detectives in discovering what an infant or toddler is revealing to us" (Gehl & Bohlander, 2018). This is a two-way street for adults and children, as adults can learn about their role as caregivers and tune in to an awareness of themselves.

Your attentiveness when parenting infants will help you both gain mindfulness. Your infant will start to learn what responses and reactions you'll give them, whether positive or negative, and, with mindful practices, you can learn how to respond appropriately without using force, yelling, or becoming frustrated in chaotic moments. Prepare to move a bit slower with your infant as not every feeding time or bath time needs to be rushed. When you slow this process down, infants will grow to learn that they can also stay calm and mindful when they finally begin completing tasks on their own.

Mindfulness for Children

Once children are old enough to attend school, they're still learning to communicate effectively and are building their vocabulary bank to do so. More distractions may arise as friendships form, but mindful skills are all the more vital here as children experience more opportunities to exert their independence from you. Once a child can communicate more clearly with their parent, it's time to discuss how mindfulness can help them in school and in life.

Talk to your child about breathing strategies, slow counting strategies, or meditation techniques that could help calm them down. While they may not want to try these at school, they can practice at home to gain control over the feelings they've experienced throughout the day. Naming any big feelings that your child has encountered also helps you connect with what they face during the day when you're not around. Discussing scenarios that they have or could possibly experience can assist them in visualizing effective strategies for self-regulation and empathy.

Mindfulness for Adults

Even as adults, we constantly work to find the right words to tell others how we feel. As a child becomes an adult, they gain the experience that helps them deal with specific situations, but some adults still resort to throwing tantrums akin to a toddler's behavior if something doesn't go their way. If they have a history of learned mindfulness, however, they'll have techniques to employ that focus on awareness, kindness, and positivity.

By the time we're adults, many of us have figured out how to communicate on a basic level, but many of us still don't know how to listen. Pausing to actively listen to others, even when they're saying something we don't want to hear, takes maturity and patience. When we're able to listen more intently, we often learn more, become more curious, and show growth in an understanding of ourselves.

As parents, encouraging children to communicate and listen well can support decision-making skills later in life as well as boost general mental wellness, so introducing these ideas to children can help create open connections (Marie, 2022). This also adds to your peace of mind as a parent, knowing that the mindful practices you've helped your child learn will continue to be methods that they can pull from when stressed or anxious.

Setting Realistic Parenting Standards

Many parents experience exchanges with their children that they're not proud off. It's important to know you're not alone here – it's not easy being a parent and there's no guidebook on how to be 'the best' parent (because there is no such thing!). Parenting is an incredibly unique experience for everyone. What is perhaps more important than being the 'perfect' parent, is to understand how you can accept the moments when you're not your best, learn from them, grow with them, and keep moving towards being a parent you can be proud of.

When you observe your child while playing or completing daily tasks, you can start to realize what mindful practices may be best for them, but it's important to also let mindfulness happen naturally rather than trying to force participation.

Setting realistic goals for children and communicating these ideas clearly with a child once they're able to understand you is one of the simplest ways to start practicing mindfulness today. For example, during mealtime, you can engage in mindful eating by taking turns describing the colors, textures, and flavors of your food without judgment. You could also practice mindful listening by sitting quietly together and focusing on the sounds around you, such as birds chirping or cars passing by. Through these practices, you can teach your children how to be present in the moment, manage their emotions, and cultivate a greater sense of calm and awareness.

Slowly introducing children to mindful practices such as guided meditation, body scanning, and deep breathing exercises can also help to calm a child's mind and offer them a fresh perspective before continuing with their day. Children enjoy a consistent routine as well, even if they don't like to admit this, so scheduling a time to meditate or simply breathe and relax before a nap or at bedtime can offer them a chance to calm their minds.

At any age, children will attempt to test their boundaries and assert their independence, so try to remain flexible as you work on mindful practices with them. Share your ideas with them, but make adjustments when needed as your child grows. You won't need to explain every detail of the benefits of mindful practices to them; simply keep the technique easy and fun so they find it enjoyable. Remember that your modeled behavior is one of the most influential tools you have when it comes to parenting, so setting a tone of appreciation for mindfulness can be the number one way to get a child eager to participate in mindful actions.

A Parent's Needs

Any person who has spent even a single day with a child can understand how important reserving self-care time can be. Since mental health connects to physical health, it's necessary to take care of your needs as well. As you know from any stress you've faced in your life, tension piles up and tends to get released in negative ways if we don't create outlets for de-stressing. Since a parent who is tired and anxious will likely not be their best self when interacting with their child, save time to meditate, walk outside, read a book, or journal your thoughts as a way to free some of the pressure you may face as a parent.

Taking Breaks

As mentioned, modeling mindful behavior for your child is one of the best ways to show your child that you respect and love yourself. Planning a night out with your friends or partner while your child has fun with a babysitter or family member lets them see that you need time for social activities just like they do.

Allow your child to see you putting your phone away and taking conscious breaks from electronic devices so they also know the time you spend with them is important. Children notice more than we think they do, and when they see a parent attached to and constantly staring at their phone, they might seek attention in any way possible, even through the use of negative means. Take breaks to dance, sing, and play with your child. They'll remember the feelings they had during these experiences with you as they get older, even if they don't remember every activity you did together.

In one study measuring emotional intelligence and the impact of device use by parents and their children ages five to twelve, researchers discovered that parents who used cell phones more frequently in front of their children had children with a lower emotional intelligence (2023):

> Parental phone use is associated with 'still face,' an expressionless appearance that's often interpreted as depression, which can further impact a child's development of emotional skills. The takeaway is for parents to be more mindful of how often they are using their phones around their children...Where their eyes are sends a message to their children about what's important. (Hamm)

Key Takeaways

Now that you're able to reflect on some of the calming mindful practices that you've pinpointed for yourself, consider how you can incorporate mindfulness while spending time with your child. Even if this simply means modeling your own mindful behavior, your child will see this and learn from your ability to self-regulate, listen, and care for yourself and others.

- Introducing mindful techniques to children can help them develop strategies to use throughout their lives.

- At any age, mindful techniques can help children develop communication skills and empathy for others.

- Parents can help children incorporate mindful breathing techniques and/or meditation into their day as well as model the importance of such practices.

- Setting realistic goals for children and remaining adaptable to any change of plans helps set the tone for mindful parenting.

- Saving time for self-care as a parent can allow you to calm your mind and take breaks.

Finally, we'll examine what it means to practice mindfulness as you age. While it's never too late or too early to start practicing mindfulness, it's meant to be a practice that's ongoing so you can enjoy the rich benefits of stress reduction.

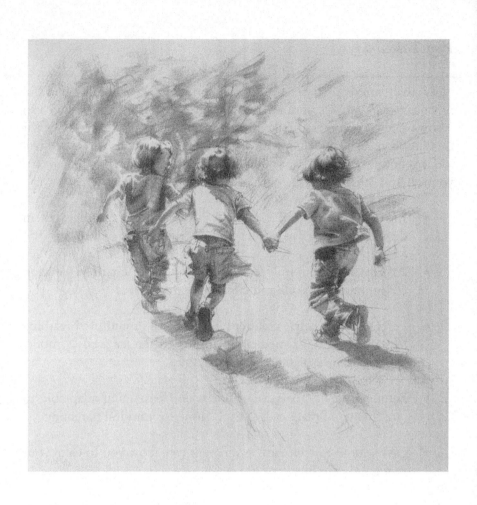

Chapter 14:

Mindfulness at Any Age

It's everywhere. When you walk into almost any store, you're likely to be inundated with gorgeous models on posters and advertisements showing what you can buy to have younger-looking skin, lose weight, or dress like a celebrity. It's hard to avoid feeling like we're not attractive enough when we live in a culture that values beauty and fears aging. While changes to a body's appearance are fairly inevitable as we get older, maintaining a mindful attitude throughout life can help us feel balanced and confident well into old age.

A Child's Mind

We know that children are impressionable and absorb ideas and lessons every day, but surprisingly, teaching mindfulness to children has only recently gained popularity in school systems. While schools and community groups are starting to pay closer attention to the advantageous impact of yoga, meditation, self-calming strategies, and deep-breathing techniques for children, the results of such practices also seem to help young children understand that there are ways to gain an awareness of their feelings without resorting to verbal or physical violence. "What research exists to date suggests that self-regulation may improve as a result of mindfulness training during childhood. In particular, mindfulness training studies with school-age children and adolescents have documented improvements on teacher and parent indices of self-regulation" (Zelazo & Lyons, 2011).

Now that you've become more aware of the positive impact mindfulness can have, consider how these practices could have benefitted you if learned in childhood. Introducing mindfulness practices to children can assist in self-management as adults. The practice of mindfulness is not valued in society nearly as much as it should be. "Mindfulness training may provide practice in reflective reprocessing...while also minimizing influences that interfere with prefrontal cortical function (e.g., cortisol/stress) and maximizing influences that promote this function (e.g., dopamine/approach-oriented emotions such as happiness and curiosity)" (Zelazo & Lyons, 2011). For a child, this means that mindful practices can help with the development of decision-making skills, problem-solving, and creativity.

Aging with Grace

As we age, it sometimes becomes more difficult to start a new hobby or gain an interest in something we've never tried before, but mindful practices tend to fit easily into a schedule and can be simple enough to practice in almost any location during your day. Keep in mind that it's never too late to begin a practice of mindfulness and that the brain benefits greatly from the continuation of learning new ideas. "Evidence suggests that meditation, prayer, and other related religious and spiritual practices may have significant effects on the aging brain—positive effects that may help improve memory and cognition, mood, and overall mental health" (Newberg, 2011).

Because we know that training the mind with puzzles, new skills, and concentration exercises can help to deter the aging process of the brain, realize that there's always room for growth and development in your life. While you may want to assume you're an expert on something you've practiced for years, break free from this fixed mindset to understand that you can always learn new ideas about a topic at any age.

When a person focuses on a realistic goal, they tend to stay motivated in achieving that outcome. As we age, we can always adapt our goals, but consider what you want to look and feel like five years, ten years, or even twenty years from now and focus on working toward goals that will help you develop your purpose. On our path toward achievement, we learn more about ourselves and others, and may even decide that we want to change our timeline or mindful exercises completely to fit our lifestyle. While focusing on the present moment is a key objective in mindful practices, planning for our future success and development can drive us in a desire to remain mindful.

Maintaining Mindfulness

Someone who isn't as familiar with the idea of mindful practices and how these can help might be under the impression that they're a waste of time or that there's too much to accomplish throughout the day to add mindful practices. They might judge some practices as being too "new age" for them when, in actuality, these practices have been benefiting individuals for centuries. While it's important to socialize and connect with others, never allow anyone to ridicule the mindful practices that help you relax or set the stage for your day.

Staying mindful means *you* control your life. You're developing the power to let ideas float to you and away from you gently and easily. The thoughts that, at one time, might have caused you stress are now simply ideas that you can observe objectively and make decisions about when the time is right. To paraphrase and apply this to the quotation mentioned earlier (in Chapter 6) from Dr Viktor Frankl, mindfulness allows you to find that space, between stimulus and response, and gives you the freedom to make your choice.

While we can't control everything that will happen in life, we can make more mindful choices to ensure we're taking care of ourselves, in both body and mind. Going to the doctor for regular check-ups, talking to your physician or therapist about any stress or concerns you're having, and planning self-care activities throughout your day are some basic ways that you can remain proactive about your well-being (Brettingen, 2022).

Of course, continuing hobbies or activities that you already participate in can keep your brain active and alert, but try branching out to find new interests that will get your mind working. Join groups that allow you to give back to your community, volunteer, and make a difference in your world. This kind of endeavor has the added benefit of helping you feel satisfied by the work you're doing and with the way you're utilizing your time. Participating in activities like this can also be a great way to meet like-minded individuals who enjoy mindful practices as much as you do!

What Your Future Holds

Since we never know for sure what our future has in store for us, it's helpful to practice healthy ways of expressing ourselves and releasing stress so we can deal with anything coming our way. We can always plan for positive outcomes with mindful practices, and stay ready for some surprises, too. If you're the type of person who enjoys staying on top of every minute of what your day will look like, adding a mindful exercise like meditating for just ten minutes can offer you a chance to escape and de-stress, while remaining open to the unknown. Suppose you're laid back and relaxed about completing tasks throughout your week. In that case, mindfulness can offer you an opportunity to appreciate and be grateful for what you have and the attitude you possess. The bottom line is that mindful practices are not for a certain *type* of person, but are for *every* person to enjoy and gain benefits from.

By treating yourself with kindness, you alter the way your brain views the world. You'll most likely notice this effect as one of the first benefits of mindful practices. Taking time out of your day to practice self-care not only gives you something to look forward to but also trains your brain to feel positive about practicing mindfulness and incorporating it into your new way of thinking. "We know anticipating something positive actually helps to maintain dopamine levels in your brain...So just the very idea of anticipating something good can physically change your brain chemistry so you feel happy" (Volpe, 2020). Start enjoying the simple moments in your life and feeling excitement about your mindful future.

Key Takeaways

Now that we're reaching the end of our exploration into the positive ways the brain can be impacted by mindfulness, I invite you to continue your understanding by applying practices and scheduling time for your mindful path. When you set a routine for mindfulness, *you* make it a priority, which will show others that you value the opportunity for mindful exercises. To further support you with this, I have included bonus content accessible from the appendix.

- Studies that measure the impact of mindfulness on school and community groups are determining that practices such as yoga, meditation, and deep breathing seem to have a positive effect on young children.

- As a person ages, mindful practices help improve and maintain memory, concentration, and self-awareness.

- Continuing to learn stimulates portions of the brain and releases healthy chemicals for more positive moods and emotions.

- Making mindful decisions for our bodies and health ensures we continue to remain proactive in caring for ourselves.

Learning anything new takes commitment and effort, but mindfulness is a practice that can become a natural way of life by simply inviting it into our day. It doesn't have to take much time from our schedule, and its effects will make us much more productive throughout the day.

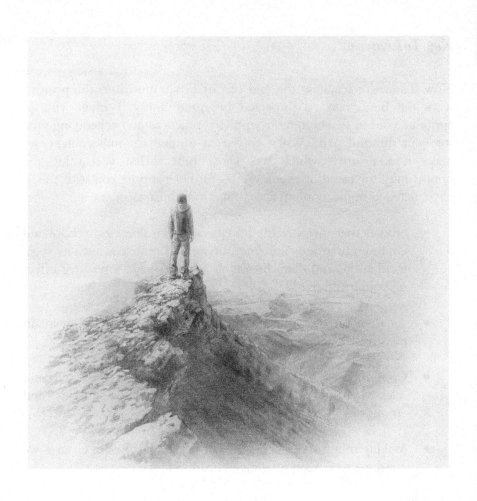

Conclusion

So often, individuals don't take the time to understand and reflect on how their lives could be improved with simple changes. I'm challenging and encouraging you today to process the work you've completed throughout this book because, whether you realize it or not, you've done a great amount already. You've taken the initiative to understand more about yourself and how to improve your brain health.

As mentioned before, if you try to take on too much at once, the effect will be minimal since you're likely to burn out quickly and return to former behaviors. Instead of trying to implement all of the ideas from this book into your life simultaneously, I'd like you to think of one practice or technique that you're going to try out today that will feel calming and beneficial for you. Because your brain, with its amazing neuroplasticity, is capable of adapting and responding in new ways, start considering techniques that can both challenge and comfort this incredible organ.

What's Next For You?

Remember that this can be your "year of mindfulness" starting now. Use the lists at the end of the chapters to settle your brain and body, and guide you into your next phase of experimentation with mindful practices. The end of this book doesn't mean the end of your mindful journey. Instead, view this as an invitation to proceed with the next steps. Through bonus content in the appendix, you're set to track your mindful adventure and begin exploring engaging exercises that can stimulate brain function and improve memory.

If you're still doubting whether you have the energy to become a more mindful person, consider this. *You* are the only one who controls your next steps. Yes, you're probably pulled in many different directions throughout your day, and balancing it all can feel difficult, but with the incorporation of mindful practices, you're likely to enjoy improved cognitive functions, a boosted immune system, and better nights of sleep to handle it all. In addition, the stress relief you experience from settling into a state of mindfulness will become more familiar to you as you continue practicing various techniques.

Your brain is a bank, and mindful practices are the small deposits you'll make that will reward you in time. Don't wait until you're stressed beyond belief to begin practicing a mindful exercise. Create mindful opportunities on the good days and the bad ones. I'm venturing to guess that you'll find benefits to experiencing calm, quiet moments on both busy and peaceful days. Consider waking each morning with the confidence to practice necessary self-care, eat mindfully, and make conscious choices daily. Mindfulness truly is life-changing and now, with help from this book, you have hundreds of ideas that you can turn to when you need a quick action to calm yourself.

Whether you're a parent who needs to recharge your energy and inspire a child with mindful practices, an athlete hoping to gain more concentration in your craft, or an employee who works hard every day wanting to feel satisfaction in your productivity, the mindful messages I'll continue to provide will allow you to enjoy new and engaging methods of mindfulness for brain health.

I'd like to kindly ask for a moment of your time. If you found value in the insights, strategies, and knowledge shared in this book, I would greatly appreciate it if you could leave a review. Your thoughts and feedback are invaluable, and I'll read all your comments and reviews. They not only inspire me to continue creating content that matters but also help fellow readers make informed decisions about their reading choices. Your review is a small gesture that can make a big impact. Thank you

I wish you positivity and progress in your continuation of what you've dared to begin. The mindful effort that you're working on now will pay off on days when you feel worn out and frustrated. On days like these, you'll know how to take the time you need to refresh your mind's energy. Enjoy this new adventure and remain open to the possibilities!

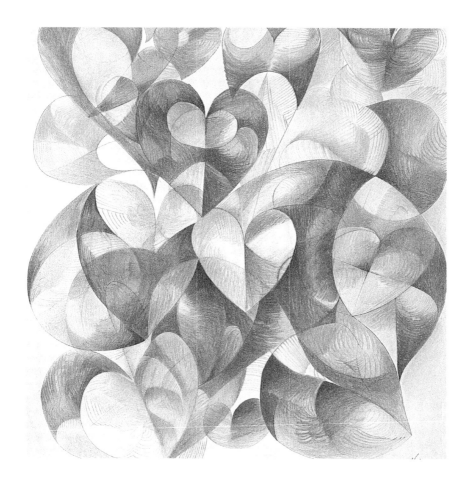

Sharing the Gift of Mindfulness

Dear Reader,

Now that you have everything you need to bring more peace into your daily life and support your brain health through mindfulness, you can help others find their path to wellbeing too. ☺

Just like focusing on your breath can create a moment of calm, your honest review on Amazon can create a ripple of positive change. **Your words could guide someone else who feels overwhelmed or stressed to discover these simple but powerful practices for themselves.**

Thank you for helping spread the message of mindfulness. When we share our experiences with others, we create a community of support and understanding – and you're helping make that possible.

Simply leave a review using the link or QR code for your Amazon marketplace

USA	UK
Amazon.com/review/create-review?&asin=1738558118	Amazon.co.uk/review/create-review?&asin=1738558118

Or search your **Local Amazon Marketplace** and enter
ASIN=1738558118
or search "Mindfulness for Brain Health by Dr Sui Wong".

With gratitude, Dr. Sui Wong

Appendix

Book Bonuses: For **FREE audioguides on guided mindfulness practices**, please register using the following link or QR code below

bit.ly/mindfulness-book-bonuses

Thursday Tips! Get my popular Thursday Tips [TT] where I share bite- size brain health tips to thrive – a 1-min read with 3 tips and 1 question! – sign up via **bit.ly/drwongbrainhealth**

Get alerts on upcoming book releases, via **bit.ly/drwongbrainhealth**

***

Other Books by Dr Sui H. Wong MD FRCP

My mission here is to write high-quality books that EMPOWER you to improve your health and wellbeing, and INSPIRE you to take action, so you can thrive and live a full and meaningful life.

***

Sleep Better to Thrive

https://books2read.com/sleepbetter

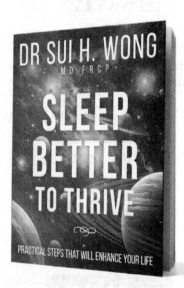

Reclaim Your Nights, Revitalize Your Days

Tired of lying awake at night? Struggling with brain fog, poor concentration, and daytime fatigue?

Sleep Better to Thrive offers a natural, holistic approach to quality sleep without relying on medications or caffeine. This practical workbook provides:

- Science-backed insights into your sleep cycles and circadian rhythm

- Simple, affordable strategies to overcome sleep disruptions

- Custom worksheets to design your perfect sleep routine

- Targeted solutions for busy families and age-related sleep challenges

More than just a sleep guide—it's a comprehensive approach to enhancing memory, mood, productivity, and long-term brain health.

Quality sleep is your brain's superpower. Are you ready to unlock it tonight?

>> GET *Sleep Better to Thrive* (available in Paperback and Kindle Unlimited, LINK: **https://books2read.com/sleepbetter**

***

Sweet Spot for Brain Health

books2read.com/sweet-spot-brain-health

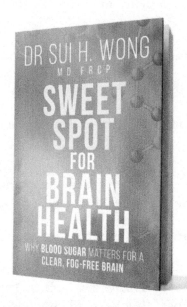

Conquer Sugar Cravings, Unlock Your Brain's Potential

Struggling with brain fog, energy crashes, and relentless sugar cravings? Your blood sugar might be sabotaging your mental clarity.

Sweet Spot for Brain Health delivers science-backed strategies to:

- Balance blood glucose naturally for sharper focus

- Harness intermittent fasting for metabolic flexibility

- Satisfy your sweet tooth without compromising health

- Implement immediate nutrition changes for lasting results

Unlike other approaches, this guide offers practical solutions that work with your lifestyle—not against it.

Includes a BONUS 12-week challenge to transform knowledge into sustainable habits.

Your brain thrives on balanced blood sugar. Are you ready to find your sweet spot?

>> GET *Sweet Spot for Brain Health* (available in Audiobook (various platforms), Paperback, Hardcover, and Kindle Unlimited, LINK: **books2read.com/sweet-spot-brain-health**

Glossary

- **Amygdala:** The small portion of the brain that assists in discerning risky situations and controlling emotions, behavior, and knowledge.

- **Body Scanning:** A mindful practice that encourages stress relief by focusing on relaxing parts of the body in a concentrated manner.

- **Brainstem:** The area of the brain that provides messages to the rest of the body since it connects the brain to the spinal cord.

- **Cerebellum:** The part of the brain that assists in muscular function and is located toward the back of the brain, near the spinal cord.

- **Cerebrum:** The largest portion of the brain that assists with functions of behavior, language, and connecting the meaning of sensory information.

- **Circadian Rhythm:** The natural body rhythm that responds to hunger, temperature, sleep cycles, and hormone release. This rhythm notes changes to surroundings throughout a 24-hour day cycle.

- **Episodic Memory:** The ability to remember particular events from the past and recall the details of the experience.

- **Frontal Cortex/Lobe:** The portion of the brain that assists with making plans and decisions based on the ability to judge situations. This portion also controls an individual's attentiveness and impulsivity.

- **Gray Matter:** The brain's neural tissue that contains fibers for processing speech, cognitive functions, movement, and bodily sensations.

- **Hippocampus:** Located in the temporal lobe, this area of the brain assists in storing memories. The hippocampus is one of the most vulnerable areas for memory loss if it's damaged due to neurological disorders or physical trauma.

- **Mindfulness:** A state of awareness that can be gained through the practice of calming activities that focus on viewing thoughts and feelings from a more objective point of view.

- **Mindfulness-Based Cognitive Training (MBCT):** A type of therapy that concentrates on mindful practices to improve awareness. This form of therapy is mainly used to treat symptoms of depression.

- **Neuroplasticity:** The brain's ability to change and rewire its synapses based on its experience of learning or adapting to situations.

- **Neurotransmitters:** The chemical released in the brain that provides information to the body's muscles and nervous system.

- **Nociception:** The nervous system's ability to process damage to body tissue or to sense extreme temperatures.

- **Occipital Lobe:** The rear portion of the brain that allows for facial recognition and visual discernment.

- **Pain Reprocessing Therapy:** A type of therapy treatment that assists in relieving chronic pain by rewiring the brain to respond differently to body pain.

- **Parietal Lobe:** The upper midsection of the brain that processes senses and outer stimuli.

- **Prefrontal Cortex:** Made up of the frontal lobe, this portion of the brain processes emotions and behavior to play a role in cognitive functions.

- **Progressive Muscle Relaxation (PMR):** A therapeutic method that helps relieve stress, headaches, digestive problems, and other chronic issues through the practice of tensing and releasing muscles throughout the body.

- **Synapse:** The small space at the end of neurons that passes messages from the brain to the nervous system.

- **Temporal Lobe:** The lower midsection of the brain that assists with language, memory, and processing emotions.

References

Note about references: This book has been written for the public. For this reason, I've decided not to limit the references to academic papers only. As such, the references and additional resources listed here include websites that you may find interesting or helpful as you go on your journey.

American Psychological Association. (2018, November 1). *Stress effects on the body*. American Psychological Association. https://www.apa.org/topics/stress/body

Ashar, Y. K., Gordon, A., Schubiner, H., Uipi, C., Knight, K., Anderson, Z., Carlisle, J., Polisky, L., Geuter, S., Flood, T. F., Kragel, P. A., Dimidjian, S., Lumley, M. A., & Wager, T. D. (2021). Effect of pain reprocessing therapy vs placebo and usual care for patients with chronic back pain. *JAMA Psychiatry*, *79*(1). https://doi.org/10.1001/jamapsychiatry.2021.2669

Atlas, L. Y., Dildine, T. C., Palacios-Barrios, E. E., Yu, Q., Reynolds, R. C., Banker, L. A., Grant, S. S., & Pine, D. S. (2022). Instructions and experiential learning have similar impacts on pain and pain-related brain responses but produce dissociations in value-based reversal learning. *ELife*, *11*, e73353. https://pubmed.ncbi.nlm.nih.gov/36317867/

Bahl, S., Milne, G. R., Ross, S. M., Mick, D. G., Grier, S. A., Chugani, S. K., Chan, S. S., Gould, S., Cho, Y.-N., Dorsey, J. D., Schindler, R. M., Murdock, M. R., & Boesen-Mariani, S. (2016). Mindfulness: Its transformative potential for consumer, societal, and environmental well-being. *Journal of Public Policy & Marketing*, *35*(2), 198–210. https://www.jstor.org/stable/44164852?read-now=1&seq=2#page_scan_tab_contents

Bargh, J. A., & Morsella, E. (2008). The unconscious mind. *Perspectives on Psychological Science*, *3*(1), 73–79. https://www.ncbi.nlm.nih.gov/pmc/articles/PMC2440575/

Barnhofer, T. (2019). Mindfulness training in the treatment of persistent depression: Can it help to reverse maladaptive plasticity? *Current Opinion in Psychology*, *28*, 262–267. https://doi.org/10.1016/j.copsyc.2019.02.007

Baron Short, E., Kose, S., Mu, Q., Borckardt, J., Newberg, A., George, M. S., & Kozel, F. A. (2010). Regional brain activation during meditation shows time and practice effects: An exploratory FMRI study. *Evidence-Based Complementary and Alternative Medicine*, *7*(1), 121–127. https://doi.org/10.1093/ecam/nem163

Batson, J. (2021). *Workplace stress - The American Institute of Stress*. The American Institute of Stress. https://www.stress.org/workplace-stress

Bernstein, A., Vago, D. R., & Barnhofer, T. (2019). Understanding mindfulness, one moment at a time: An introduction to the special issue. *Current Opinion in Psychology*, *28*, vi–x. https://doi.org/10.1016/j.copsyc.2019.08.001

Brahm Centre. (2020, August 31). *Neuroplasticity - how mindfulness reshapes the brain | Dr Sara Lazar*. Youtube.com. https://www.youtube.com/watch?v=wP9X6QIaflU

Boys Town National Hotline. (n.d.). *10 ways to stay grounded*. Your Life Your Voice. Retrieved January 17, 2024, from https://www.yourlifeyourvoice.org/pages/10-ways-to-stay-grounded.aspx

Brahm Centre. (2020, August 31). *Neuroplasticity - how mindfulness reshapes the brain | Dr Sara Lazar*. Youtube.com. https://www.youtube.com/watch?v=wP9X6QIaflU

Brettingen, P. J. (2022, August 30). *How to age gracefully by changing your mindset*. DailyOM. https://www.dailyom.com/journal/how-to-age-gracefully-by-changing-your-mindset/

Broadway, K. (2023, May 25). *The benefits of mindfulness for student-athletes | NCSA.* Ncsasports.org. https://www.ncsasports.org/blog/benefits-of-mindfulness-for-athletes

Brown, K. W., Goodman, R. J., Ryan, R. M., & Anālayo, B. (2016). Mindfulness enhances episodic memory performance: Evidence from a multimethod investigation. *PLOS ONE*, *11*(4), e0153309. https://doi.org/10.1371/journal.pone.0153309

Campbell, L. (2016, May 17). *Personal boundaries: Types and how to set them.* Psych Central. https://psychcentral.com/relationships/what-are-personal-boundaries-how-do-i-get-some

Celestine, N. (2020, August 15). *What is mindful breathing? Exercises, scripts and videos.* PositivePsychology.com. https://positivepsychology.com/mindful-breathing/

Corporate Wellness Magazine. (n.d.). *Workplace stress: A silent killer of employee health and productivity.* Corporatewellnessmagazine.com. https://www.corporatewellnessmagazine.com/article/workplace-stress-silent-killer-employee-health-productivity

Cunningham, C., Kashino, M. M., & Phillips, H. G. (2018, January 18). *10 easy ways to make your home more peaceful.* Washingtonian. https://www.washingtonian.com/2018/01/18/10-easy-ways-to-make-your-home-more-peaceful/

Damasio, A. R. (1999). How the brain creates the mind. *Scientific American*, *281*(6), 112–117. https://www.jstor.org/stable/26058529

Dobbs, I. (2018, March 4). *Neuroplasticity.* Science for Sport. https://www.scienceforsport.com/neuroplasticity

Dunne, J. D., Thompson, E., & Schooler, J. (2019). Mindful meta-awareness: Sustained and non-propositional. *Current Opinion in Psychology*, *28*, 307–311. https://doi.org/10.1016/j.copsyc.2019.07.003

Eby, S. (2023, June 5). *Hydration tips for athletes | Mass general Brigham.* Massgeneralbrigham.org. https://www.massgeneralbrigham.org/en/about/newsroom/articles/tips-for-staying-hydrated

Garey, J. (2023, November 6). *Practice mindful parenting | mindfulness techniques.* Child Mind Institute. https://childmind.org/article/mindful-parenting-2/

Gehl, M., & Bohlander, A. H. (2018). Being present: Mindfulness in infant and toddler settings. *YC Young Children, 73*(1), 90–92. https://www.jstor.org/stable/90019488

Giles, J. (2019). Relevance of the no-self theory in contemporary mindfulness. *Current Opinion in Psychology, 28*, 298–301. https://doi.org/10.1016/j.copsyc.2019.03.016

Grant, J. A., & Zeidan, F. (2019). Employing pain and mindfulness to understand consciousness: A symbiotic relationship. *Current Opinion in Psychology, 28*, 192–197. https://doi.org/10.1016/j.copsyc.2018.12.025

Hamm, K (2023, March 23). How parents' smartphone use affects their kids. https://www.universityofcalifornia.edu/news/how-parents-smartphone-use-affects-their-kids

Hartfiel, N., Havenhand, J., Khalsa, S. B., Clarke, G., & Krayer, A. (2011). The effectiveness of yoga for the improvement of well-being and resilience to stress in the workplace. *Scandinavian Journal of Work, Environment & Health, 37*(1), 70–76. https://www.jstor.org/stable/40967889

Harvard School of Public Health. (2020, September 14). *Mindful eating.* The Nutrition Source. https://www.hsph.harvard.edu/nutritionsource/mindful-eating/

Harvard T.H. Chan School of Public Health. (2019, August 21). *Packing a healthy lunchbox.* The Nutrition Source.

https://www.hsph.harvard.edu/nutritionsource/kids-healthy-lunchbox-guide

Henriksen, K. (2022). The magic of mindfulness in sport. *Frontiers for Young Minds, 10.* https://doi.org/10.3389/frym.2022.683827

Herz, R. (2016). The role of odor-evoked memory in psychological and physiological health. *Brain Sciences, 6*(3), 22. https://doi.org/10.3390/brainsci6030022

Hölzel, B. K., Carmody, J., Vangel, M., Congleton, C., Yerramsetti, S. M., Gard, T., & Lazar, S. W. (2011). Mindfulness practice leads to increases in regional brain gray matter density. *Psychiatry Research: Neuroimaging, 191*(1), 36–43. https://doi.org/10.1016/j.pscychresns.2010.08.006

Hölzel, B. K., Lazar, S. W., Gard, T., Schuman-Olivier, Z., Vago, D. R., & Ott, U. (2011). How does mindfulness meditation work? Proposing mechanisms of action from a conceptual and neural perspective. *Perspectives on Psychological Science, 6*(6), 537–559. https://www.jstor.org/stable/41613530

Hougaard, R., & Carter, J. (2016, March 4). *How to practice mindfulness throughout your work day.* Harvard Business Review. https://hbr.org/2016/03/how-to-practice-mindfulness-throughout-your-work-day

Ivey, P., McGuire, R., & Lattner, A. (2015, July 29). *Mind over matter.* Training & Conditioning. https://training-conditioning.com/article/mind-over-matter-d36/

Jiménez-Picón, N., Romero-Martín, M., Ponce-Blandón, J. A., Ramirez-Baena, L., Palomo-Lara, J. C., & Gómez-Salgado, J. (2021). The relationship between mindfulness and emotional intelligence as a protective factor for healthcare professionals: Systematic review. *International Journal of Environmental Research and Public Health, 18*(10), 5491. https://doi.org/10.3390/ijerph18105491

Johns Hopkins Medicine. (2022). *Brain anatomy and how the brain works.* Hopkinsmedicine.org. https://www.hopkinsmedicine.org/health/conditions-and-diseases/anatomy-of-the-brain

Kabat-Zinn, J. (1994). *Wherever you go, there you are: Mindfulness meditation in everyday life.* Hyperion.

Kabat-Zinn, J. (2013). *Full catastrophe living: Using the wisdom of your body and mind to face stress, pain, and illness.* Bantam Books.

Katella, K. (2022, May 31). *How to be more resilient: 8 strategies for difficult times.* Yale Medicine. https://www.yalemedicine.org/news/resilience-strategies-pandemic

Kraemer, K. M., Jain, F. A., Mehta, D. H., & Fricchione, G. L. (2022). Meditative and mindfulness-focused interventions in neurology: Principles, science, and patient selection. *Seminars in Neurology, 42*(02), 123–135. https://doi.org/10.1055/s-0042-1742287

Kylie, U. (2018, February 22). *The unconscious brain - finding clarity during unconsciousness.* Michiganmedicine.org. https://www.michiganmedicine.org/health-lab/what-happens-brain-during-unconsciousness

Maldonado, K. A., & Alsayouri, K. (2023). *Physiology, brain.* PubMed; StatPearls Publishing. https://www.ncbi.nlm.nih.gov/books/NBK551718/

Marie, S. (2022, March 25). *All about mindful parenting.* Psych Central. https://psychcentral.com/health/mindful-parenting#definition

Mayo Clinic. (2021, February 4). *Traumatic brain injury - symptoms and causes.* Mayo Clinic. https://www.mayoclinic.org/diseases-conditions/traumatic-brain-injury/symptoms-causes/syc-20378557

Mayo Clinic. (2021, March 24). *Stress management.* Mayo Clinic; Mayo Clinic. https://www.mayoclinic.org/healthy-lifestyle/stress-management/in-depth/stress-symptoms/art-20050987

Miller, J. (2014). Roll model: a step-by-step guide to erase pain, improve mobility, and live better in your body. Victory Belt Publishing

Miller, J. (2023). Body by breath: the science and practice of physical and emotional resilience. Victory Belt Publishing.

Newberg, A. B. (2011). Spirituality and the aging brain. *Generations: Journal of the American Society on Aging, 35*(2), 83–91. https://www.jstor.org/stable/26555779

Pacheco, D., & Callender, E. (2021, January 15). *Bedtime routines for children.* Sleep Foundation. https://www.sleepfoundation.org/children-and-sleep/bedtime-routine

Puderbaugh, M., & Emmady, P. D. (2023). *Neuroplasticity.* PubMed; StatPearls Publishing. https://www.ncbi.nlm.nih.gov/books/NBK557811/

R. Morgan Griffin. (2010, May 11). *10 health problems related to stress that you can fix.* WebMD; WebMD. https://www.webmd.com/balance/stress-management/features/10-fixable-stress-related-health-problems

Raio, C. M., Orederu, T. A., Palazzolo, L., Shurick, A. A., & Phelps, E. A. (2013). Cognitive emotion regulation fails the stress test. *Proceedings of the National Academy of Sciences, 110*(37), 15139–15144. https://doi.org/10.1073/pnas.1305706110

Regan, S. (2023, July 26). *21 grounding techniques to try the next time you feel stressed out.* Mindbodygreen. https://www.mindbodygreen.com/articles/how-to-ground-yourself

Reid, M. C., Eccleston, C., & Pillemer, K. (2015). Management of chronic pain in older adults. *BMJ: British Medical Journal, 350.* https://www.jstor.org/stable/26518254

Rupprecht, S., Koole, W., Chaskalson, M., Tamdjidi, C., & West, M. (2019). Running too far ahead? Towards a broader understanding of mindfulness in organisations. *Current Opinion in Psychology, 28,* 32–36. https://doi.org/10.1016/j.copsyc.2018.10.007

Segal, Z. V., Williams, J. M. G., & Teasdale, J. D. (2002). Mindfulness-based cognitive therapy for depression: A new approach to preventing relapse. Guilford Press.

Segal, J., Smith, M., Robinson, L., & Shubin, J. (2023, February 28). *Improving emotional intelligence (EQ).* HelpGuide. https://www.helpguide.org/articles/mental-health/emotional-intelligence-eq.htm

Semeco, A. (2017). *20 simple ways to fall asleep as fast as possible.* Healthline. https://www.healthline.com/nutrition/ways-to-fall-asleep

Sevinc G, Hölzel BK, Hashmi J, Greenberg J, McCallister A, Treadway M, Schneider ML, Dusek JA, Carmody J, Lazar SW (2018). Common and Dissociable Neural Activity After Mindfulness-Based Stress Reduction and Relaxation Response Programs. Psychosom Med, 80(5):439-451. doi: 10.1097/PSY.0000000000000590.

Sivadas, A., & Broadie, K. (2020). How does my brain communicate with my body? *Frontiers for Young Minds, 8*(540970). https://doi.org/10.3389/frym.2020.540970

Straw, E. (2023, May 29). *Visualization techniques for athletes-Success starts within.* Successsstartswithin.com. https://www.successsstartswithin.com/blog/visualization-techniques-for-athletes

Tang, Y.-Y. ., Lu, Q., Fan, M., Yang, Y., & Posner, M. I. (2012). Mechanisms of white matter changes induced by meditation.

Proceedings of the National Academy of Sciences, 109(26), 10570–10574. https://doi.org/10.1073/pnas.1207817109

Toussaint, L., Nguyen, Q. A., Roettger, C., Dixon, K., Offenbächer, M., Kohls, N., Hirsch, J., & Sirois, F. (2021). Effectiveness of progressive muscle relaxation, deep breathing, and guided imagery in promoting psychological and physiological states of relaxation. *Evidence-Based Complementary and Alternative Medicine, 2021*(1), 1–8. https://doi.org/10.1155/2021/5924040

Valluri, J., Gorton, K., & Schmer, C. (2024). Global meditation practices: A literature review. *Holistic Nursing Practice, 38*(1), 32–40. https://doi.org/10.1097/HNP.0000000000000626

Volpe, A. (2020, December 29). *Science says you need to plan some things to look forward to.* Vice.com. https://www.vice.com/en/article/7k9wvb/science-says-you-need-future-plans-to-look-forward-to-during-pandemic

Walker, M. P. (2006). Sleep to remember: The brain needs sleep before and after learning new things, regardless of the type of memory. naps can help, but caffeine isn't an effective substitute. *American Scientist, 94*(4), 326–333. https://www.jstor.org/stable/27858801

Walker, M. P. (2018). *Why we sleep.* Penguin Books.

Wein, H. (2021, March 29). *Good sleep for good health.* NIH News in Health. https://newsinhealth.nih.gov/2021/04/good-sleep-good-health

Wong SH, Pontillo G, Kanber B, Prados F, Wingrove J, Yiannakas M, Davagnanam I, Gandini Wheeler-Kingshott CAM, Toosy AT (2024). Visual Snow Syndrome Improves With Modulation of Resting-State Functional MRI Connectivity After Mindfulness-Based Cognitive Therapy: An Open-Label Feasibility Study. J Neuroophthalmol, 44(1):112-118. doi: 10.1097/WNO.0000000000002013

Zelazo, P. D., & Lyons, K. E. (2011). Mindfulness training in childhood. *Human Development, 54*(2), 61–65. https://www.jstor.org/stable/26764991

Images Reference

I created the illustrations at the end of each chapter using Midjourney **www.midjourney.com** and am grateful for this tool that helped me bring forth my vision for these images.

Made in the USA
Las Vegas, NV
11 May 2025

21984470R00105